PROGRAMMING YOUR LIFE WITH AYURVEDA

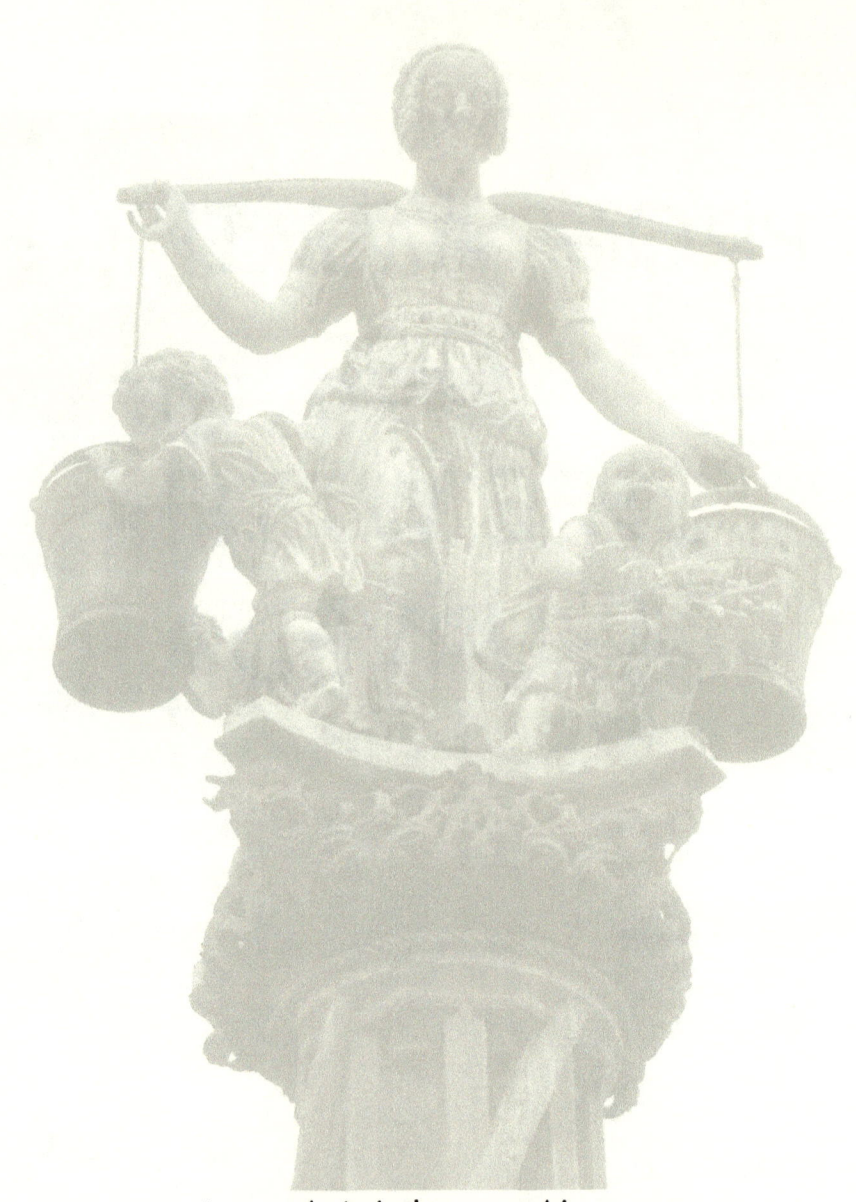

Ayurveda is balance and harmony

Dr. Vinod Verma

PROGRAMMING YOUR LIFE WITH AYURVEDA

A practical manual for a holistic way of
living for well being, health,
and preventing ailments

Gayatri Books International

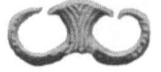

The information provided in this book is not intended to replace the services of a physician. The suggestions for a healthy way of living with Ayurvedic life-style provided in this book are for the purpose of self-help and education. The author and the publisher are in no way responsible for any medical claims regarding the material presented in this book. For using methods and remedies provided in this book at commercial level requires the prior permission from the author. For more information, write to the author directly at ayurvedavv@yahoo.com

Translation rights are with the author. The book is already published in German, French, English, Slovenian, Czech and Hindi. Write to the author directly at ayurvedavv@yahoo.com
or ayurvedavv@gmail.com for translation rights.

Visit Dr. Vinod Verma at www.ayurvedavv.com and www.drvinodverma.com to find out about her seminars, lectures and consultations, etc. Information is also provided at the back pages of the book.

ISBN: 978-1495243332

Dedication

This book is dedicated to my Guru, Acharya Priya Vrat Sharma who always imparted generously from his immense wisdom of Ayurveda and Indian tradition. My dedication is also to my students and readers from all over the world who have been a constant source of inspiration through their feedback.

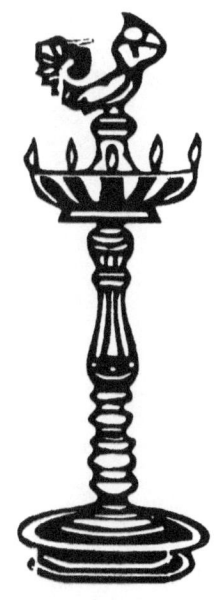

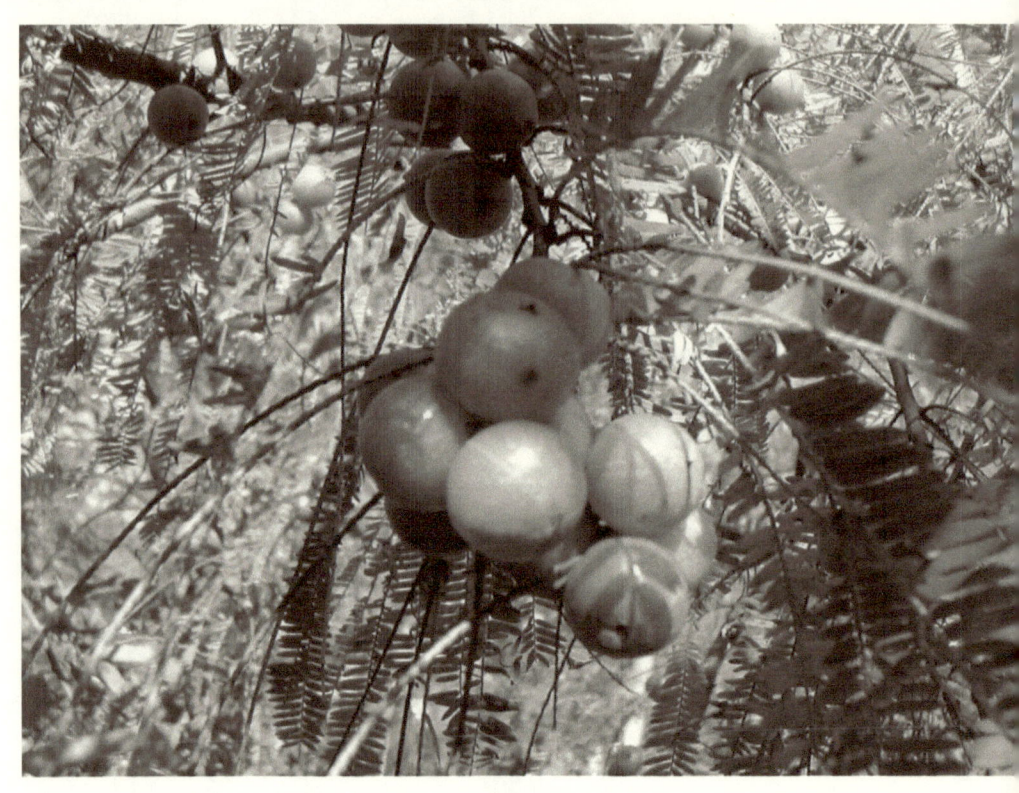

Amala

Foreword

Ayurveda is not only a system of medicine but also primarily discusses life and life processes aimed at longevity and improving the quality of life to maintain and make it happy and wholesome. I have summed up my view in the following shloka for defining Ayurveda:

आयुः सुखं हितंदीर्घ येन विन्दति मानवश्व
आयुषन्च परिज्ञान मायुर्वेदः स उच्यते॥

'Ayurveda is that which imparts knowledge about life and all its aspects and by which a human being attains happy, wholesome and long life.'

Thus, one can shape an ideal lifestyle by following the guidance prescribed in Ayurveda. In other words, Ayurveda can be utilised as the best guide to improve and formulate a lifestyle so as to make it fit and suitable to the circumstances. In today's world, it has become more important to save oneself from the pressure generated from stress and strain caused by the environmental conditions.

Dr. Vinod Verma has rightly chosen this topic and has discusses the subject in a masterly manner. She has already written a dozen books on various aspects of Ayurveda, which have become popular. I congratulate Dr. Verma for this opportune and valuable contribution.

Professor Priya Vrat Sharma
Gurudham, Varanasi
10th October, 2003

Preface

This book is a practical manual with demonstrative pictures and it is written on the demand of my students. Through my books, lectures, and seminars in Europe and at my two centres in India, the practical wisdom of Ayurveda (what I also call 'grandmother's tradition of Ayurveda') is imparted. This practical guide will be beneficial for those who wish to adopt Ayurvedic practices for health and harmony and also for those who have attended my seminars but did not get any practical training in my centres. This book is meant to initiate you into Ayurvedic way of living and thinking in order to fight back the unhealthy ways of stress and strains the modern society imposes upon us. In my previous books, I have presented my aphoristic interpretation of the Ayurvedic texts:

"The first priority of life is life itself"

Give it a thought and make the best out of your precious life span. What matters more than the 'quantity' of life in terms of years, is the 'quality' of life. By 'quality of life' I do not only mean that one should be free of disorders and ailments and attain vigour and vitality. It also means a peaceful mental state and wisdom to keep a balance during the ups and downs of life. It is to attain the mental strength to face life with dignity and courage and to discover your spiritual strength through sattva— the inner stillness of the mind. Ayurveda is science of life and it deals with every aspect of our day-to-day life. It is a very expansive subject and that is the reason that I have devoted my life writing on various dimensions and aspects of Ayurveda. This particular book is essentially a practical manual to integrate Ayurvedic practices in your everyday life. Wherever necessary, I have given the appropriate references from my other books.

Food is a very important aspect of Ayurvedic living and it is a subject that has to be dealt with in detail. I have, therefore, written a separate book, called *Ayurveda Food Culture and Recipes* (available at www.amazon.com).

I suggest that you go through the whole book first and then try to assimilate one by one the practices given here in your daily routine. Try this new way of life to break your current mechanical routine. You will soon realise a change occurring in your looks as well as in your energy level.

You will need to devote sometime in the beginning to study and understand the basics of Ayurvedic system and the way of living. Follow then the programmes step by step. You will realise that gradually, these will become a part of your routine and you will follow it quite spontaneously. You will soon learn to observe your body functions and will be able to cure your minor discomforts and ailments. In fact, it is the accumulation and persistence of smaller disorders, which ultimately give rise to serious diseases. Therefore, this small investment in terms of your time for purifying your mind and body will be highly beneficial in the long run.

In the first Chapter, I have given a very simple introduction to the principles of Ayurveda. I have specially dealt with the questions most commonly asked by the beginners. The urban Indians and foreigners largely think that Ayurveda is an ancient system of medicine, and when they think of medicine, their reference frame is modern medicine (also called allopathy). The allopathic system treats human body like a machine that can be analysed in terms of its parts. This is a reductionist approach where both time and matter can be reduced to smaller units. In fact, many modern writers, particularly western, have also approached Ayurveda in a similar manner. Ayurveda is not merely a system of medicine; it is also a systematic treatise on the way of life to enhance energy and prevent ailments. It is not possible to approach this holistic system of life in a fragmented manner. Ayurveda recognises that the physical, mental, social, philosophical, spiritual and cosmic dimensions of our being are interrelated, interconnected and interdependent. Your stomach problems may originate from simply a bad sitting posture or anger or excessive worry. In such cases, medication, appropriate diet, yoga asanas and counselling are required simultaneously. Similarly, persisting constipation or partial evacuation will lead to a series of ailments over a period of time and also gives rise to bad dreams, dull and drab complexion, menstrual pains, and so on. This book is meant to create awareness in you for a holistic way of life, so that you are able to see the interrelationship and interdependence of various aspects of your being.

The simple Ayurvedic practices given in this book will get you initiated into a healthy living and will improve the quality of your life by enhancing your immunity and vitality (called ojas in Ayurveda). Once you adopt this lifestyle and see the results, you will get curious to learn more from this ancient wisdom.

The wisdom provided in this book is gathered from varied sources ranging from Atharva Veda to the living tradition of India in different parts of the country. Whatever the sources, the collected information has been constantly subjected to research for its effectiveness, and additions and new discoveries have been made. This book is the result of my fourteen years of teaching yoga and Ayurveda for good health and preventing ailments. My constant interaction with students has enabled me to make this systematic yet simple treatise on the daily practices of Ayurveda. Fourteen years ago, it would not have been possible for me to write this book as my mind was then bubbling with the academic and scriptural wisdom of Ayurveda. This wisdom is absolutely essential to understand the living tradition of Ayurveda. Living traditions are mostly the simplified and practicable versions of the academic wisdom and in the renaissance of Ayurveda; many try to impose the academic wisdom on the home-wisdom, which is neither appropriate nor practical.

I have made a special effort in this book to take into consideration the constraints of modern life with its hectic pace and stress. My suggestion is that you give your health a priority over your other activities and think of investing in your old age just as you invest money for your future. Good luck!

Vinod Verma
August, 2000
www.ayurvedavv.com

Present revised edition

This book was written thirteen years ago and has been worldwide appreciated for being extremely practical for adopting Ayurvedic lifestyle. It has been translated into German, French, Czech, Slovenian and Hindi. The present edition is being presented in the same form with minor alterations. Hope the younger generation will be able to benefit from it the same way. As said earlier, this book is not for learning the profound aspects of Ayurveda, but its practice in daily life. Once the reader benefits from the practices, can get interested to learn the subject more profoundly and related books are referred.

I wish you all good health and high quality of fulfilled life!

Vinod Verma
ayurvedavv@yahoo.com
www.ayurvedavv.com   www.drvinodverma.com

January 2014

Acknowledgements

Programming your life with Ayurveda is the result of more than a decade of teaching 'Ayurveda in everyday life' or 'Ayurveda, a way of life'. The wisdom compiled in this book is a long-term study on Ayurvedic practices used in the folklore tradition, as well as in classical Ayurveda. As I was teaching, I went on adding some new practices. Based upon the principles of Ayurveda, I invented some practices which are easy to do for people on their own— like for the replacement of 'nasya', the classical Ayurvedic practice for the purification of the head region. I am grateful to all my students for their feedback and to those people who brought me data from different folkloric practices.

Our Vedas and Charaka Samhita have immense wisdom that can guide us for keeping good health and maintaining mental equilibrium. My guru, Acharya Priya Vrat Sharma has done tremendous amount of research work to translate and compile four volumes of Charaka Samhita. Dr. Satvelakar's translation of the Vedas is unparallel. Thus, I am indebted to ancient sages as well as the sages of our times for providing this wisdom to us.

I am grateful to my editor Mahendra Kulshreshtha for going through this book with care and for his valuable editorial suggestions.

I am indebted to my nieces and nephews for modelling. Most pictures given in this book are from Gayatri and Abhinav while Shruti and Pranav also participated in this venture.

'A right minded person with intellect, potency and prowess should look for his well-being, here and in the world hereafter; should pursue three desires such as desire for life, desire for wealth and desire for the other world.

Out of all these desires, one should follow the desire to live first. Why? Because on departure of life, everything departs. Life should be maintained by observing the code of conduct for the healthy and being prompt in alleviating disorders.

Next to life, it is wealth that is to be sought. There is no bigger curse than to have a long life without means (to sustain it).'

Charaka Samhita Sutrasthana
600 BC

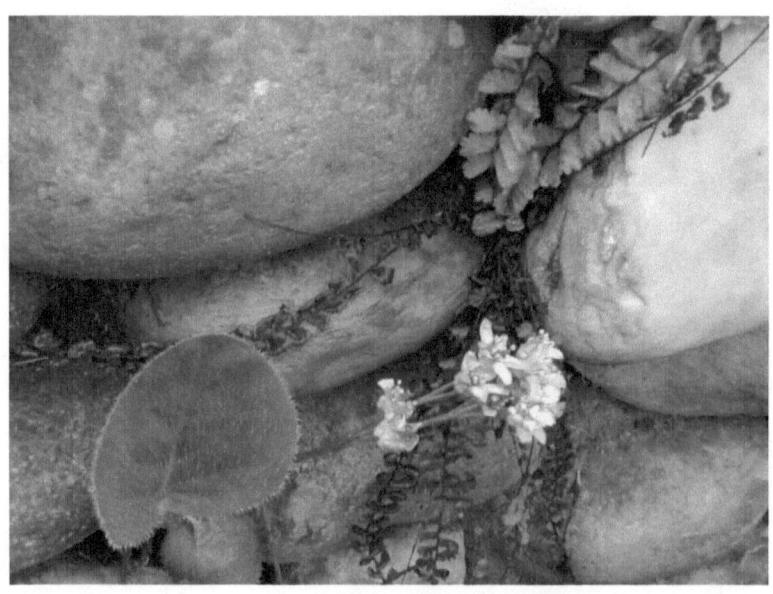

Contents

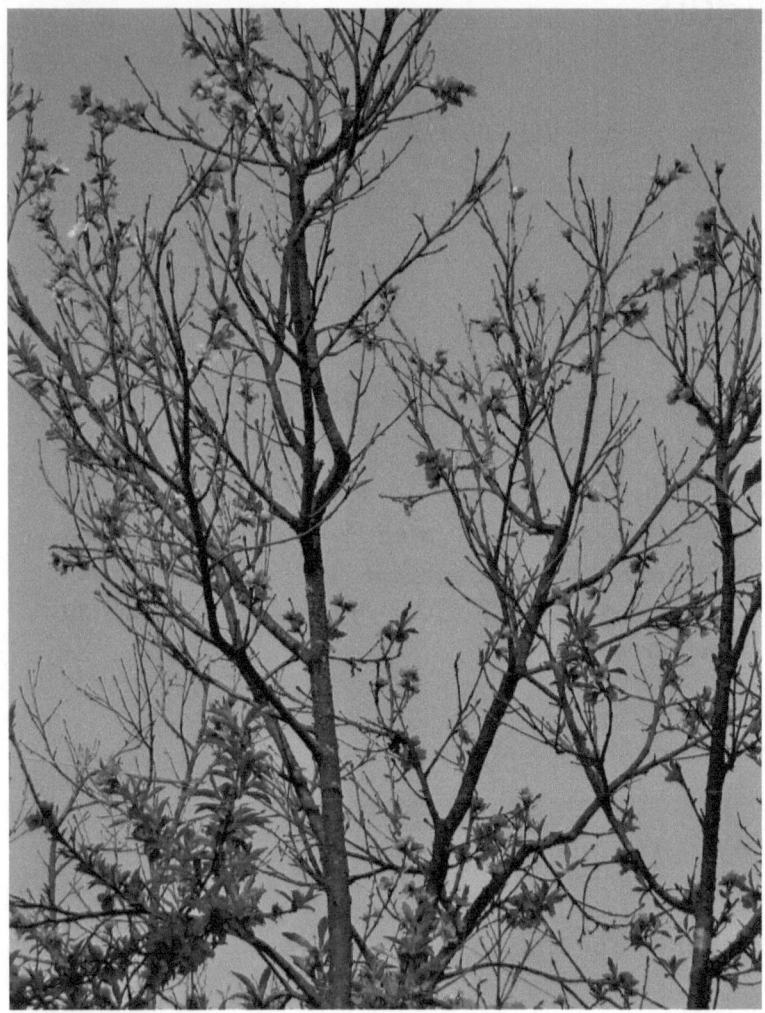

Shirish tree

Chapter 1

Introduction to Ayurveda

Ayurveda is the wisdom about life from ancient India. Some call it 'the science of life'. Ayurveda tells us the art as well as the craft of living. When there are hindrances like mental or physical pain, disorders, ailments and diseases, it provides remedies for them and prescribes methods to bring the body to equilibrium and harmony again. Ayurveda also includes the science of rejuvenation in order to enhance vitality and minimise the effects of ageing. Ayurveda is not merely a medical system from ancient India as is understood by many. It is a comprehensive science of life that also provides suggestions about how to live an enriched, happy and disease-free life and how to enhance the pleasures of life. It also instructs on optimising the quality of life and enhancing one's life span. All this is not only done with remedies of natural origin and balanced nutrition but also with one's mental and spiritual efforts. The word '*Ayus*' means life or duration of life (the time between birth and death) and *Veda* means wisdom. Thus, this scriptural wisdom deals with the totality of life with reference to individual needs relating to physical and mental health, family structure, social situations, environment, and spiritual development.

History of Ayurveda

It is said that Ayurveda is as ancient as humanity itself and that Lord Brahma started this tradition while he created the universe. In any case, the first written documentation about Ayurveda is from Rig Veda and Atharva Veda. Recent research shows that the Vedas are between 3500 to 5000 years old. The oral tradition of the Vedas is yet more ancient than this period. Rig Veda is the most ancient of all the four Vedas. After the Rig Veda, Yajur and Sam Vedas were composed and Atharva Veda is the last of the four Vedas. In Rig Veda, there are various references to the medicinal and healing arts whereas Atharva Veda (the Veda of fire) is the source book of Ayurveda from ancient India. It is not exclusively a treatise on medicine as it also deals with other aspects of life such as material, social, political, ritualistic and so on. It is in Atharva Veda that we find the first reference to the three principal energies of the body—the vata, pitta and kapha. Atharva Veda also talks about spiritual healing through various ceremonies. Use of spiritual therapy along with rational is greatly emphasised in Atharva Veda and it is a very impressive documentation from the ancient world which reveals three-dimensional holistic therapy— rational, psychological and spiritual. The rational therapy was done with drugs made from plants or minerals, the psychological therapy was done through rituals and ceremonies with repetitive mantras and spiritual therapy was done mostly through the worship of the cosmic powers like the sun, moon, trees, mountains, rivers, etc. It may be for fighting an infection or a smooth childbirth or attracting the mind of a lady towards you; Atharva Veda is enriched with ceremonious methods for all these. Healing plants are treated with respect and gratitude is shown towards them. The following is said about our most familiar kitchen spice, curcuma or turmeric (*haldi*), which has also become famous in the world now:

Full of vitality, oh *Haridre!* (curcuma), you are the best of all medicines, like the sun and the moon during the day and the night respectively. (Atharva Veda, VI, 29).

In Atharva Veda, there are groupings of medicinal plants for curing various skin ailments (I, 24). There are descriptions of diseases like hepatitis, malaria, typhoid, tuberculosis, epilepsy, etc., and also there are anatomical details of the human body. I have discussed this subject in more detail in my book, *Ayurveda, A Way of Life*. I mention some of these here as I have been very much inspired by this Veda and the spiritual dimension of Ayurvedic programmes described in this book is the result of my research on this valuable ancient book and its utilisation in our daily lives.

Later on in history, Ayurveda was compiled as a separate Veda from the four ancient Vedas. The most complete and detailed text we possess on Ayurveda, written at least one thousand years later than the Atharva Veda is *Charaka Samhita*. The basic concepts of *Charaka*

Samhita were formulated by sage Atreya around 1000 BC. Atreya developed these by discussing different themes of Ayurveda with scholars and sages in various symposia organised in different parts of the country. The most brilliant of his disciples was Agnivesha who documented these in the form of a treatise called *Agnivesha Tantra*. About three centuries later, this text was enlarged and refined by Charaka and it came to be known as *Charaka Samhita*. Around 4 AD, Dridhabala rewrote *Charaka Samhita* by making many additions from relevant materials available at that time and it is his edition that we have at present.

Another important school of Ayurveda from ancient India is that of Dhanvantari which probably was at the same time as Atreya. But this was exclusively a surgical school. The text available from this school is *Sushruta Samhita* compiled by the great physician and surgeon Sushruta who was a contemporary of Charaka. *Sushruta Samhita* is a valuable text because in addition to medicine, it describes techniques of surgery, rhinoplasty and has details of surgical instruments.

Ashatanga Samgraha and *Ashatanga Hridaya* were written by Vagbhata in 6 AD. He summarised the views of Charaka and Sushruta and added original scientific data concerning the treatment of diseases.

I do not want to go into the details of historical accounts here. However, it is important to mention that in addition to the healthy way of living, principles of general medicine and surgery, the ancient Ayurvedic literature describes eight different specialities:

1. Internal medicine
2. Paediatrics
3. Diseases related to eyes, ears, nose and throat
4. Psychiatry
5. Surgery and rhinoplasty
6. Toxicology
7. Rejuvenation and longevity
8. Virility, sexuality and fertility

Ayurveda was always developed and expanded and it has always been part of the living tradition of India. During the Muslim expansion, it was transported to Baghdad where it contributed to the Unani system of medicine. In modern times, Ayurvedic wisdom has contributed to allopathy and homeopathy.

In *Charaka Samhita*, there are descriptions of the environment, the quality of water and air and vitiation in weather, climate, etc. due to the degradation of environment. Since in a holistic system, everything is interrelated and interdependent, the degradation of environment, change in weather and climate and other such factors are extremely important. It is said that the food and medicines grown in the degraded environment are likely to lose their effectiveness resulting in the derangement of all life.

The extensive wisdom of *Charaka Samhita* is beyond space and time and we should benefit from it. Unfortunately, many people, both at home and abroad, think that Ayurveda is just about some prescriptions to cure various physical ailments. The next theme will further clarify this misconception.

Is Ayurveda Scientific?

Ayurveda has become popular throughout the world during the last decade. I recall when I did research for my book *Ayurveda, A Way of Life* in the late eighties; I was hesitant to use the Sanskrit terminology for the English and German editions that appeared in 1992. But now there are many Panchakarma centres in Germany and Switzerland and the words panchakarma, abhiyanga, shirodhara etc., have become household words there. Ayurveda is not a recognised medical system in the West, yet it is extensively used for prevention and relief. In the West, other systems of medicine, whether they are from the East or of their own alternative methods of healing from the Middle Ages, are not recognised as scientific.

The western medical conception of 'scientific' is within the narrow precepts of the reductionist approach to Science that is discussed in the next topic. According to it, ailments should be technically detectable and measurable and drugs should be standardised on laboratory animals and through clinical studies. Individual human constitution and circumstances are not taken into consideration. The Ayurvedic view of looking at health, disease and treatment differs in its fundamental approach but it should not mean that it is not scientific.

Many people in the world confuse Ayurveda with herbal medicine or other similar methods of healing. Herbal medicine or many other healing methods from folklore traditions of the world are prescriptions of certain plant medicines for ailments or are descriptions of the other methods or ceremonies for healing. They are not complete scientific systems like Ayurveda where the aetiology of diseases, pharmacology of the medicinal substances, doses, toxicology, nutrition in relation to time, place and special circumstances, surgery, psychology, psychiatry, social behaviour and responsibilities of physician as well as patients and hundreds of other related themes are described. In Ayurveda, it is advised that rational, mental and spiritual therapies should be applied simultaneously and not independent of each other. I cite below the views of Acharya Priya Vrat Sharma on the holistic and scientific approach of *Charaka Samhita* from his Introduction of Charaka Samhita's translation:

The law of uniformity of nature was established which helped in applying the physical laws to the biological field. It remains a mystery for all in what type of laboratories and with what equipment they were able to arrive at these scientific truths. Perhaps the entire nature was their laboratory and their own keen observations and divine vision worked as their instruments.

...In order to stabilise the idea (of rationality), 'yukti' was added to one of the pramanas (means of valid knowledge). Charaka has emphasised all through to work according to yukti (rationale). He has advised to move always with knowledge. There should be a proper correlation of theoretical knowledge (jnana) and practical skill (karma). Charaka has emphasised on the process of investigation which is essential for arriving at scientific truths...
...For advanced knowledge and research, they adopted the method of discussion amongst experts. Symposia were organised in different parts of the country in which experts of the subject participated.

...Charaka Samhita holds the synthetic view of man instead of analysing him as aggregates of tiny cells. Happiness and unhappiness are final consequence of health and disease respectively and these affect the person wholly and not partly. Tri

dosa, as well as the psyche pervade the whole body and therefore in health and disease.... this deha-manasa (body-mind) approach is a very important contribution of Charaka Samhita in the field of medicine.

...Man is not a machine and as such can't be operated equally with a uniform law. Every person has got his own individuality and normal variations. This forms his constitution which distinguishes him from other individuals. This is termed as 'Prakriti'. Every regimen or therapy has to be applied keeping in view the constitution of the concerned person and his suitability.

In the *Encyclopaedia Britannica*, Science is described as follows: 'Any of the intellectual activities concerned with the physical world and its phenomena and entailing unbiased observations and systematic experimentation. In general, a science involves a pursuit of knowledge covering general truths or the operations of fundamental laws.'

Let us consider the above statements which Acharyaji has given with the light of the way modern science is defined in the West. Ayurvedic wisdom is 'intellectual activities concerned with the physical world and its phenomena and entailing unbiased observations and systematic experimentation'. Besides that, knowledge and wisdom of Ayurveda, has stood the test of thousands of years and its validity is beyond space and time.

Many people think that Ayurveda propagates ahimsa (non-violence) and suggests a vegetarian diet or is associated with some religion, and so on. These are absolutely false notions, and reasons for these are that many a times Ayurveda is brought to the West through religious gurus and it is tinged with sects or religions and with their own specific interpretations. *Charaka Samhita* has the description of all kinds of meats and wines. It is about nature and the natural ways of building strength, healing and therapy. Study of *Charaka Samhita* reveals that it does not have any moral, religious or philosophical bias. However, compared to the western scientific wisdom, Ayurveda has different fundamental principles and these are based on the uniformity of the cosmos and the cosmos being a dynamic whole.

Mechanistic versus Holistic

Since most of you who will read or use the wisdom in this book may be influenced by modern medicine (allopathy), it is important that I point out here the basic difference in the approach of these two systems. Modern medicine is based upon the concept that the cosmic reality is material and that it can be approached with the senses. The material reality can be split into further fragments up to atoms and so on. Both, the cosmos and the human body work like a machine and time is conceived as linear. This 19th century notion of Western physics is still applied in modern biology and medicine. Disease, health and other events in life are dependent on chance factors. Contrary to it, the Ayurvedic approach is that the cosmos is a dynamic, ever-changing whole where every function is for a definite purpose, where time is cyclic and it is a perfected system that works on cause, effect and its substratum. We human beings are a part of this large system in which our dynamic bodies and minds form a smaller system. All systems, smaller and bigger, are interconnected, interrelated and interdependent. The physical and sensual reality is only one dimension of the multi-layered reality.

In modern medicine, ailments and disorders are recognised with their objective and measurable symptoms and thus treatment is given on the basis of these symptoms. The human body is compared to a machine that can be analysed in terms of its parts. Discomfort or illness is seen as the malfunctioning of the body-machine. Different mechanisms of the body are understood at biological and molecular levels and disorders are treated with physical or chemical intervention. For the purpose of treatment, body and mind are considered as separate entities. Both time and matter are reduced to smaller units and chance plays an important role in causing malfunctions and disorders.

Contrary to the above views, in the holistic system of Ayurveda, an individual is considered as a non-divisible unity, an integral whole which cannot be reduced in terms of its parts, nor can the individual be separated from the social, cultural and spiritual environment and the cosmic link. An illness is viewed as the consequence of disharmony with the cosmic order. It does not occur by chance and it is not limited in space and time. Matter is interlinked, interconnected, interdependent and dynamic and it is this transformation that denotes time. Time is not linear but cyclic. For understanding malfunctions and for treatment, the social, cultural and spiritual environments of an individual are taken into consideration.

Let me give you a simple example to elucidate the above statements. Constipation or partial evacuation is considered a very minor disorder in the allopathic system. It is due to wrong food, lack of movements or diminished motility of the intestines. It should be treated by removing its causes and with some chemical intervention.

In Ayurveda, besides the above-mentioned causes, constipation may be due to fear, insecurity or a hectic way of life. It is extremely important to evacuate well and twice a day. Constipation or partial evacuation will lead to disturbed sleep, dry skin, pimples, headaches and nervousness. It may cause infertility and pain during intercourse. Over a long period of time, constipation may give rise to disorders like haemorrhoids, colitis and serious sleep problems. It disturbs one of the three principal energies of the body called vata. When vata is disturbed, various other disorders related to this energy may also occur. Thus, according to Ayurveda, one should ensure proper evacuation to avoid a series of ailments. Drinking hot water, relaxation, massage, specific yogic exercises, treatment with some herbs and attaining stillness of mind with various meditative methods are recommended to completely eradicate this problem.

The above example shows that when something in the body or mind is disturbed, it causes disturbance in the whole system. It causes a kind of disruption in the natural order of the system. All physical and mental functions of the body are part of a well-organised system and we should attend to it that this system does not divert from its natural order. It is the responsibility of each individual to do everything to maintain this order. When this order remains disturbed and is not attended to, it gives rise to minor ailments in the beginning, which may take a serious turn in the long run. This idea will be clearer to you after the following topics that deal with the three principal energies of the body and six dimensions of our being.

Let me give you here, in brief, some concrete principles of Ayurveda and an outline of its practical aspects.

The Three Principal Energies of the Body:
Vata, Pitta and Kapha

The story of Ayurveda begins with the five fundamental elements or *mahabhuta* that form the material reality of the universe. These elements are ether, air, fire, water and earth. The equilibrium of the five elements is essential for cosmic harmony and their imbalance and vitiation cause catastrophes in the world. Vitiation may be in the form of fast winds, fire accidents, too much heat, floods, earthquakes, etc.

Since all what exists is made of the five elements, the same cosmic principles apply to all, including human body. But the body has soul in it, which is the cause of consciousness and makes it a vital organism. For the performance of vital functions, the five elements form three principal vital energies, translated also as humours in English (*dosha* in Sanskrit). These are called vata, pitta and kapha. Vata is from ether and air, pitta is from fire and kapha is from water and earth (Figure 1). These energies perform various mental and physical functions of the body and the nature of those functions depends upon the nature of the element or elements they originate from.

Vata is responsible for entire body movements, blood circulation, respiration, excretion, speech, sensations, touch, hearing, feelings like fear, anxiety, grief, enthusiasm, etc., natural urges, formation of foetus, sexual act and retention.

Pitta is responsible for vision, hunger, thirst, heat regulation, softness, lustre, cheerfulness, intellect and sexual vigour.

Kapha constitutes the solid structure of the body and is responsible for binding, firmness, heaviness, sexual potency, strength, forbearance and restraint.

Figure 1. Three principal energies or doshas from five fundamental elements

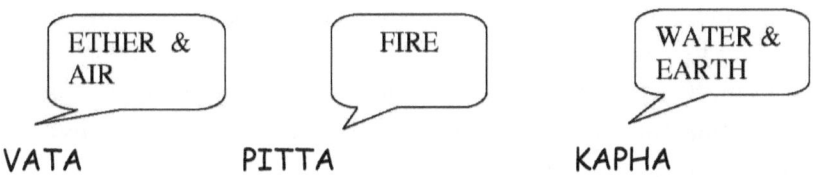

ETHER & AIR	FIRE	WATER & EARTH
VATA	PITTA	KAPHA

People differ from one another because of a slight difference in their fundamental constitution called prakriti. This difference is due to the variation in the proportion of the three main energies. This variation is in terms of dominance of a particular energy or the combination of two energies. This is what makes us different from one another and unlike machines, as the system of modern medicine tends to see us. Prakriti not only describes the variations in physiological features and reactions of individuals but also their personality types. The fundamental constitution of an individual is a very important theme of Ayurvedic wisdom for diagnosis and therapy. I have given some details of it below. For more details, consult my book, *Ayurveda: A Way of Life.* In the next chapter, very simple and practical ways of determining your prakriti are given.

For good health and a long life, these three vital forces or doshas should be in a state of equilibrium within their individual organisation as well as with respect to each other. However, if there is disturbance in one dosha and it deviates from its quality, quantity or place or if the three doshas are not in balance with each other, it leads to *vikriti* or a state of vitiation or disharmony, giving rise to diverse discomforts. Prakriti of an individual is his or her body's basic nature or fundamental constitution and the tendency of the nature is to be orderly and healthy. Due to external factors like weather, climate, stress, wrong nutrition, and so on, prakriti may change into vikriti or vitiation, which is a state of non-health. The nature of the body is such that it reverts back to its natural conditions on its own. But if the factors disturbing this nature are very strong and constantly oppress it, the state of vikriti prolongs. We need appropriate food, drugs and other measures to revert back to prakriti. However, if the state of vitiation is left unattended for a long time, it will give rise to serious disorders.

PRAKRITI OR THE INDIVIDUAL CONSTITUTION

A mother observes differences in the personality traits of her babies from the beginning and the siblings differ in their likes and dislikes of food, their reaction to weather and climate, the effect of drugs, the fundamental way of reacting to situations and other personality traits. According to Ayurveda, each one of us has an individual constitution from birth. It is the basis of our physiological and psychological reactions. For maintaining good health, it is essential to take the individual constitution into consideration.

The prakriti of an individual is due to the dominance of one or more doshas and attributes the characteristics of that particular dosha in slightly more predominance than the others. For example, the pitta prakriti individuals are sensitive to heat, sweat a lot and eat and drink in plenty. The vata prakriti ones are agile and swift in their movements. The kapha prakriti persons are slow and stable in their movements and are more tolerant than the previous two. In the mixed prakriti, the person may experience different attributes at different times and in different situations.

Seven Types of Prakriti

1. VATA   2. PITTA   3. KAPHA

4. VATA–PITTA   5. PITTA-KAPHA 6. VATA–KAPHA
7. SAMADOSHA *(all doshas in equal proportions)*

The difference in the proportions of the three energies or doshas is one factor of variation and their degree is another. For example, one may be vata dominating in varying degrees. The proportion of the two doshas may differ in the mixed prakriti. The fundamental presence of the intensity of each of the three energies is another varying factor. For example, there are some individuals with plenty of energy, tremendous stamina and vitality, very good immune system and a brilliant mind. There are others who come in a medium category whereas there are still others who are healthy but are low in their energy, stamina and mental capabilities.

Imagine the presence of the three energies in different individuals on a scale of 1 to 10. We begin at 0.1 with all the gradations up to number 10. We get 100 different cases and then we multiply them with seven types of prakriti, we will get a large number of human types. Furthermore, if we consider also the degree of dominance and in mixed prakriti, the proportion of the two doshas, we will end up with numerous sorts of prakriti.

Importance of Prakriti

Since everything in this cosmos is made of five elements including our body and everything is interconnected and interdependent, the outer factors influence us constantly. To maintain the equilibrium of the five elements in the body, which are present in the form of three energies, it is essential that an individual knows his or her constitution. If a person with a predominant fire element (pitta prakriti) does actions or consumes food with a dominance of the same element, he or she may end up getting this energy vitiated and may fall ill. Therefore, for nutrition, for maintaining health as well as for remedies, it is essential to know one's prakriti or the fundamental constitution.

The basic human nature does not change, the variations may occur due to life-situations. Imagine someone of pitta disposition who is impatient and gets angry very quickly, and has also a pitta-dominating partner. This couple may have fights, confrontations and disputes. Being similar, both these individuals will tend to enhance and aggravate each other's anger. Later on in life, imagine one of them living with a kapha-predominant person with patience and tolerance. Gradually, this pitta-dominant person will lessen his anger. The other person's patience gives time to think and reflect and not to react.

Besides being important for health and healing, the knowledge of prakriti can lead us to a better understanding of each other in family life, at work and in other aspects of social interaction.

In Tables 1-3, I have given some details about the three principal energies. There are characteristics of a dominating dosha, the factors which may vitiate it, symptoms of vitiation and corresponding remedies. These Tables are from my book *Ayurveda, A Way of Life*. These Tables give you an idea how prakriti is constantly being affected by internal and external forces. We have to learn to create an equilibrium and to counteract those forces which adversely affect our equilibrium. Windy and stormy weather can cause imbalance of vata. If we take measures like massage, fomentation, specific nutritional supplements like ginger, garlic, fenugreek, *ajwain* and other vata reducing products, the effect of windy weather will be counterbalanced. Similarly, excess of heat can cause an imbalance of pitta. Cold bath, cooling ointments like sandalwood paste, yellow earth (*Multani mitti*), cool rooms and nutrients

28

containing sweet, bitter and astringent rasas can help reduce the effect of heat on us and save us from pitta vitiation. Humid and cold weather tends to vitiate kapha. A vapour bath or hot bath, spicy meals and some exercise will counteract the effect of the weather and prevent any kapha vitiation.

There are also other factors like the time of the day, age and climate at a particular geographical location. These factors are summed up in Table 4.

Table 1. The origin, functions and characteristics of vata.

Origin and function

Vata is light, subtle, mobile, dry, cold, rough and all pervasive, like the basic elements air and ether from which it is made of and it is responsible for body movements and mind activities, blood circulation, respiration, excretion, speech, sensation, touch, hearing, feelings like fear, grief, anxiety, enthusiasm, etc., natural urges, the formation of foetus, the sexual act and its duration.

Characteristics of vata prakriti persons

*Agile, *Quick and unrestricted in their movements, *Swift in action, *Quick in fear and other emotions, *Get easily irritated, *Intolerant to cold and shiver easily, *Coarse hairs and nails, *Dry skin, *Prominent blood vessels.

Vata promoting factors

*Fasting, *Excessive physical exercise, *Exposure to cold, *Laziness, *Staying awake late at night, *Windy weather, *Old age, *Evening and last part of the night, *Over-ripened or stale foods, *Injury, *Blood loss, *Excessive sexual intercourse, *Uneven posture, *Suppression of natural urges, *Anxiety, *Guilt.

Signs of vata vikriti

*Stiffness and pain in the body, *Bad taste and dryness in mouth, *Lack of appetite, *Stomach-ache, *Dry skin, *Fatigue, *Dark coloured stool, *Insomnia, *Pain in the temporal region, *Giddiness, *Tremors, *Yawning, *Hiccups, *Malaise, *Delirium, *Dull complexion, *Withdrawn and timid behaviour.

Treatment of vata vikriti

*Food dominating in sweet and sour rasa, *Hot therapeutic measures, *Enemas, *Massages, *Anointing, *Appropriate rest, relaxation and sleep, *peaceful atmosphere, Cheerful mental state, Treatment with diet and drug.

Table 2. The origin, functions and characteristics of pitta.

Origin and Function

Pitta is hot like the basic element fire from which it is constituted. Its characteristics are sharp, sour and pungent, and it has a fleshy smell. It is responsible for vision, digestion, hunger, thirst, heat regulation, softness and lustre, cheerfulness, intellect and sexual vigour.

Persons of pitta prakriti

*Intolerant to heat, *Have a hot face and body, *Delicate organs, *Tendency to have moles, freckles and pimples, *Lustrous complexion, *Plenty of hunger and thirst, *Oily skin, *Early appearance of wrinkles, *Falling and greying hairs. *Body smell, *Intolerance and lack of endurance.

Pitta promoting factors

*Sharp, alkaline and salty foods, *Foods and drinks that give burning sensation, *Sun bathing, *Noon time, *Midnight, *Summer, *Process of digestion, *Youth, *Anger

Signs of pitta vikriti

*Excessive perspiration, *Body smell, *Abnormal hunger and thirst, *Inflammation, *Tearing and thickening of skin, *Rash, *Acne, *Herpes, *Excessive heat in the body, *Burning sensation, *Loss of contentment, *Anger, *Discontentment

Treatment of pitta vikriti

*Food dominating in sweet, bitter and astringent rasa, *Cold measures, *Unction with cooling products, *Purgation, *Fasting, *Cold baths and massage with cooling oils, *Consolation, *Treatment with diet and drug

Table 3. The origin, functions and characteristics of kapha.

Origin and function

Kapha is derived from the fundamental elements earth and water and like these elements it is soft, solid, dull, sweet, heavy, cold, slimy, unctuous and immobile. It constitutes the solid structure of the body and is responsible for unctuousness, binding, firmness, heaviness, strength, forbearance, restraint, absence of greed and sexual secretions as well as sexual potency.

Persons of kapha prakriti

*Dull in activities, diet and speech, *Delayed initiation, *Disorderly, *Stable movements, *Well united and strong ligaments, *Cold and moist skin, *Little hunger and perspiration, *Clear eyes, face and complexion

Kapha promoting factors

*Sweet and salty foods, *Oily, fatty and heavy to digest nutrients, *Sedentary lifestyle, *Lack of body movements, *Day dreaming, *Childhood, *Spring season, *Morning time, *First part of the night

Signs of kapha vikriti

*Drowsiness, *excessive sleep, *Sweet taste in mouth, *Excessive salivation, *Heaviness in the body, *Cold sensation, *Nausea, *Itchy feeling in the throat, *Whiteness in eyes, urine and faeces, *Deformed body organs, *Weariness, *Lassitude, *Inertness and depression

Treatment of kapha vikriti

*Foods dominating in pungent, bitter and astringent rasa, *Hot and rough measures, *Pressure massage, *Wet heat, *Vamana or voluntary vomiting, *Physical activities, *Reduced sleep, *Treatment with diet and drug

Table 4. Relationship of the time of the day, age and climate to human constitution or prakriti

DOSHA	TIME	AGE	CLIMATE
KAPHA	Morning Evening	Childhood	Humid cold
PITTA	Noon Midnight	Youth	Dry hot
VATA	Afternoon Night	Middle-age and old age	Dry cold Windy

Note: The hot and humid climate is pitta-kapha promoting.

The Three Characteristics of Mind

Time, place, situation, nutrition, emotions, etc. constantly influence our doshas or the vital forces and by learning about the influence of these factors on your particular constitution, you can learn to maintain the equilibrium. The three vital forces (vata, pitta, kapha) are also related to our thought process and therefore it is essential to maintain an equilibrium in the three characteristics of the mind, which are:

1. Rajas
2. Sattva
3. Tamas

The rajas includes thinking, planning and taking decisions. The tamas is that which hinders motion (like state of sleep, fatigue or laziness) and expansion of the mind (emotions like greed, anger, jealousy, and so on).

The sattva includes equilibrium, goodness, truth, compassion, stillness and peace. An imbalance of sattva, rajas and tamas not only influences the equilibrium of the humours but also causes mental ailments. Thus, for maintaining good health and preventing ailments, a six dimensional equilibrium is essential as the three dimensions at two levels influence each other. Imbalance of the three characteristics of mind influences the equilibrium of doshas and vice versa.

The Six-Dimensional Equilibrium

Our state of mind influences our principal energies (vata, pitta and kapha), which are responsible for the physical and mental functions of the body. For example, if we are worried or are over-worked or have excessive mental stress, vata gets vitiated and some symptoms of its vikriti appear (see Table 1). Too much anger influences pitta and one can suffer from pitta-related disorders like stomach ailments (see Table 2). Depression gives rise to kapha-related disorders leading to obesity, nausea, excessive salivation, and so on (see Table 3).

When a vital energy is in a state of imbalance and there are related disorders, they in turn influence the mental state of an individual. If constipation or partial evacuation persists, it can give rise to sleep disorders or a hectic mental state or nervous behaviour. Stomach problems, which are due to pitta disturbances, may enhance anger and irritation.

Thus, it is important to understand that in Ayurveda, for keeping the basic equilibrium of the body, a six dimensional effort is required. One cannot think of doing everything relating to the three doshas and expect to be in a perfect health. Equally important is to maintain a mental level of equilibrium with happiness and satisfaction. Charaka lays a great emphasis on sattva to maintain the balance between activities (rajas) and non-activities (tamas). In practice, sattva is to maintain stillness and peace of mind in diverse situations in life. Sattva is the inner light that shows us ways for various activities of life, gives us peaceful and restful sleep and helps maintain an equilibrium of the body and the mind. Santosha or a state of satisfaction is one aspect of sattva and according to Charaka, asantosha or a state of dissatisfaction is one of the principal causes of ailments.

You will see that in the Ayurveda programme given in this book, there are several exercises and activities for your daily routine which are designed to direct your life towards sattva.

Figure 2. The six dimensional equilibrium.

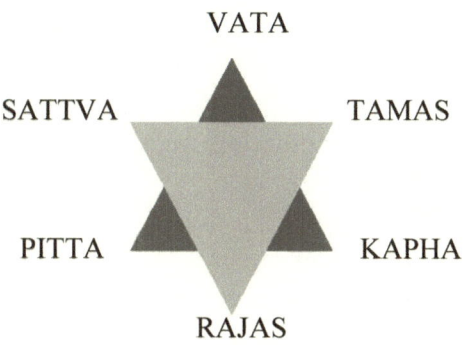

Prakriti and Vikriti

For a better understanding of the Ayurvedic principles it is very important to comprehend the dynamism of our body system and that of the cosmos. Prakriti means nature and in Ayurveda, it refers to a person's individual nature, i.e. the individual constitution in terms of the physiological and psychological personality of an individual. According to natural cosmic principles, the nature of the body is to be healthy. The individual variations account for the diversity in nature of different persons. The basic equilibrium of the three energies should be maintained for health and harmony. Since this equilibrium is constantly influenced by external factors like weather, climate, place, time (age, time of the day, time of the year) and it may be disturbed and take the form of vikriti (state of non-health), our effort should be directed to regain the state of prakriti. With knowledge and through personal effort, we can bring ourselves to the state of prakriti again. However, if the state of non-health is allowed to persist, it gradually creates severe imbalance in the body and over a period of time, there arise one or more disorders.

According to Ayurveda, one should make the best of one's efforts to prevent ailments and disorders. Despite all efforts, if there are health problems, they should be treated in a holistic manner through the three-dimensional therapy of Ayurveda (rational, mental and spiritual) and after the ailment is cured, the balance should be re-established with appropriate medication. After treatment, the patient should be given rasayanas (the health-promoting preparations) to rebuild the immunity and vitality of the body.

Ayurvedic Nutrition

Nutrition plays an extremely important role in healing as well as making people sick. We observe that millions of people around the world are over-fed and obese and suffer from various ailments due to malnutrition in the sense of excessive nutrition. Contrary to this, in the Southern Hemisphere of the globe, there are droughts, hunger, wars and famine and many people suffer from malnutrition in the sense of under-nutrition. The nutrients can be healing or poisonous for us depending on time and need. For example, after sweating a lot in heat or otherwise, if you get pain in your legs and feet, simply drinking some salted water with lemon and sugar will be an effective remedy. The same preparation will have a negative effect on someone who does not do hard work and sweats or is suffering from hypertension or diabetes. Cold milk is good for persons with pitta prakriti and during summer months. Cold milk taken by a person of kapha prakriti during winter nights can cause kapha vikriti.

There are detailed specifications in Ayurveda for nutrients and their effect on our bodies in reference to health and healing. With Ayurvedic wisdom about nutrition, one can treat oneself to get back the lost balance and regain the state of prakriti.

PRINCIPLES OF AYURVEDIC NUTRITION

The Basic Equilibrium of Nutrition and the Doshas

The body as well as nutrients are made of five elements. In the body, the five elements constitute three principal energies or doshas that perform all physical and mental functions of the body. In the nutrients, there are six principal *rasas* or tastes, which are derived from two ele ments each. Through nutrients, we supply the body with elements which in turn form the three principle energies (vata, pitta and kapha). We need the supply of these three energies constantly in our bodies as they are also consumed for performing various functions. This idea has been summarised in Figure 3.

Figure 3. The journey of the food in the body

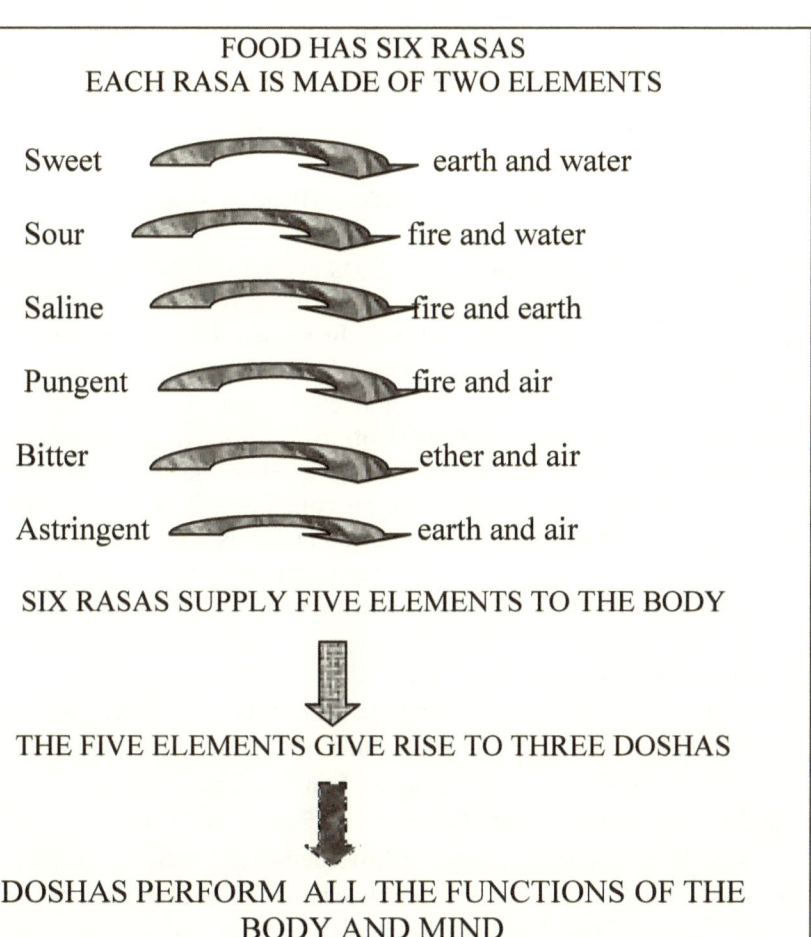

FOOD HAS SIX RASAS
EACH RASA IS MADE OF TWO ELEMENTS

Sweet — earth and water

Sour — fire and water

Saline — fire and earth

Pungent — fire and air

Bitter — ether and air

Astringent — earth and air

SIX RASAS SUPPLY FIVE ELEMENTS TO THE BODY

THE FIVE ELEMENTS GIVE RISE TO THREE DOSHAS

DOSHAS PERFORM ALL THE FUNCTIONS OF THE
BODY AND MIND

Table 5. The Relationships of the Rasas and the Doshas

DOSHA	Promoting rasas	Pacifying rasas
VATA	Pungent, Bitter, Astringent	Sweet, Sour. Saline
PITTA	Sour, Saline, Pungent	Sweet, Bitter, Astringent
KAPHA	Sweet, Sour, Saline	Pungent, Bitter, Astringent

Nutrition according to prakriti, time and space

Individuals with different constitutions need to lay emphasis on different kinds of foods. In the living tradition of Ayurveda, this aspect is dealt with in a very simple manner. In respect to their Ayurvedic nature, nutrients are either cold, hot or in equilibrium. Combinations of cold and hot create balance. The nutrients which are in equilibrium are easy to digest and are health promoting. In order to maintain an equilibrium, nutrients which are extremely cold or extremely hot in their Ayurvedic properties should only be consumed if prepared with specific spices or if eaten together with other foods with the opposite Ayurvedic properties. Ayurveda also recommends that a range of antagonist nutrients be strictly avoided (see Tables 6-7).

There is another category of internal factors which originate from the state of mind. Emotions like worry, fear, excitement, etc., may cause an imbalance of vata; anger may cause imbalance of pitta and depression may give rise to an imbalance of kapha. Thus, one should choose food according to the specific circumstances in order to maintain equilibrium. If someone is already a little depressed and eats sweet, cold, heavy and oily diet, this will enhance his/her problems. Eating in a state of anger gives rise to pitta related disorders. Take a light diet after the suppression of anger. The emotional state of mind which leads to vata imbalance should be appeased with sweet, warm and unctuous diet.

Nutrition should co-ordinate with the time of the day, the time of the year, one's age and geographical location. These are the external factors that influence the balance of our vital energies (see Table 4).

It is not possible to put the enormous wisdom of Ayurveda in just one book. I suggest that for more details on nutrition, you consult my books, *Ayurveda for Life: Nutrition, Sexual Energy and Healing* and *Ayurvedic Food Culture and Recipes*. The present book introduces you to the day-to-day practical wisdom of Ayurveda.

A few important rules regarding nutrition should always be followed:

- never eat antagonistic foods, eat heavy to digest foods only in small quantity,
- eat more of balanced foods, and
- eat very 'hot' or very 'cold' foods only in appropriate combinations.

See tables 6-7 for the Ayurvedic properties of some food products.

Quality and Quantity of Food

The food should be prepared with fresh products grown or produced in appropriate environments. It should be prepared with feelings of love, indulgence and with sattvic thoughts. If the person preparing food has tamasic thoughts like anger, jealousy, greed, etc., the prepared food carries further the tamasic energy.

One should always use aesthetic tableware and kitchen utensils and meals should always be eaten in a peaceful atmosphere and relaxed mental state. Aesthetic equipment does not mean that you should eat in silver plates or expensive crockery. South Indians serve in a wonderfully aesthetic manner on banana leaves. Simple earthenware can also be bought in beautiful forms and shapes.

Table 6. Classification of major food products according to their cold, hot or balanced Ayurvedic nature

FOODS COLD IN NATURE

Grains	Wheat, rice, maize (promotes vata), barley (increases vata), common millet and Italian millet (enhances vata), masoor beans (also called red lentils) (promotes vata), young green peas, ripe green peas (strongly vata promoting), chick peas
Vegetables	Spinach, cabbage and Brussels sprouts (vata), okra, green beans, bitter gourd (Karela), endives, fennel, aubergine, onion, celery, cucumber, beetroot, sweet paprika (without seeds), dandelion, asparagus
Fruit	Apples (sweet), bananas, pears, apricot, guava, muskmelon, water melon, figs
Dairy Products	Milk, ghee, butter
Meat	Frog, seafood, sea fish, mutton
Herbs and Spices	Clove, coriander, fennel, anise, dill leaves (not the seeds), liquorice
Others	Sugar

FOODS HOT IN NATURE

Grains	Urad beans, soya beans
Vegetables	cress salad, potatoes, cauliflower, tomatoes
Fruits	Oranges, grapefruit, lemon, grapes (which are not absolutely sweet), peaches, plums, kiwis (specially the black seeds in kiwi), nuts (almonds, peanuts, hazelnuts, walnuts, pine nuts and others), sour apples
Dairy Products	Yoghurt, processed cheese
Meat	Pork, horse, beef, freshwater fish

| Herbs and Spices | Greater cardamom, cumin, cinnamon, black pepper or white pepper, fenugreek, kalonji, garlic, basil, dill seeds, ajwain, mustard seeds, nutmeg, mint |
| Others | Honey, vegetable oils, eggs (hen, fish) |

FOODS WITH NATURAL EQUILIBRIUM

Grains	Finger millet, mung beans, chick peas at the beginning of germination
Vegetables	Carrots, turnips, small radishes (not over-ripe), zucchini, pumpkin (just ripened)
Fruits	Sweet mangoes, papaya, pomegranate, grapes (sweet)
Meat	Deer, goat, chicken
Herbs and Spices	Small cardamom, ginger, Turmeric or cur-cuma

Table 7. List of heavy to digest and antagonist foods, which may lead to imbalance

HEAVY TO DIGEST FOODS

Vegetarian foods: Urd beans, over-ripe peas, animal or plant fat, nuts or preparation from nuts, any vegetable or fruit or a preparation of food that has an extreme taste like sour, sweet, pungent, bitter, astringent, salty and when consumed in excess, raw or over-ripe vegetables and fruits, yoghurt when eaten several times a day and specially at night

Non-vegetarian foods: Pork, beef, meat of animals kept under stressful conditions, animal fat or foods containing animal fat in larger quantities.

ANTAGONISTIC FOOD COMBINATIONS

• Milk in combination with sour foods, radish, water melon or fish.
• Honey in any heated form or taking a hot drink immediately after taking honey
• Fatty food in combination with cold drinks or cold water
• Use of diet adverse to a person's food habits
• Combination of too hot and too cold foods
• Food antagonism to time, place and constitution
• Foods excessively dominating in one particular rasa like excessively salty, sweet, sour etc.

To bring oneself to a peaceful mental state, one should say a little prayer or do some breathing exercises before beginning the meal. One should get out of the physical and mental activity, bring oneself to a state of calmness and then begin to eat. Your body and mind should come to what I call, 'eating mode'. Imagine that you are cooking and going around preparing several things to have a meal ready. When the meal is ready, you want to sit and eat. Your whole being is still in activity. You need to let yourself loose. Just with five deep breaths your body and mind come to a state of relaxation. In a relaxed state, the stomach does its optimum work of digestion and assimilation. Needless to say, you should never eat anything while walking or standing.

It can be observed that many people in this world make themselves sick merely by eating too much or too many times. The stomach should never be filled more than two thirds. That means, you should never consume food to the full capacity of your stomach. According to Ayurveda, during digestion, all the three doshas are required and one should leave 1/3 space for them. If we fill the stomach to its optimum capacity, the doshas are pushed out and their vitiation takes place. It is interesting that one of my German students told me a German saying that reveals the same idea— 'leave one fourth of your stomach for the doctor'.

After every meal, one should give the stomach a rest of four hours. One should eat nothing between meals. The process of digestion takes about three hours and your stomach should get a rest of one hour. According to Ayurveda, eating before the previous meal is completely digested is detrimental to your health. If it is done frequently, it causes a serious stomach ailment. Thus, one should be very careful and eat two main meals and two small meals in a day. In between these meals, one should not eat anything. Even for a small quantity of food, the stomach has to undergo the whole process of digestion.

Purification of the Body and the Mind

In Ayurvedic wisdom, it is believed that accumulation of dirt whether externally or internally, makes the body functions sluggish and gives rise to imbalance of doshas or vital energy. All these lead to various malfunctions and ailments. It is extremely important to clean and purify the body externally as well as internally. In the course of this book, you will see that in the practice of Ayurveda, there are many methods of cleaning each and every individual parts of the body and insure their hygiene and proper functioning. During bath, it is important to clean and rejuvenate the body by scrubbing and massaging. Cleaning of the nostrils is extremely essential to ensure the unhindered passage of the air. The simplest of the inner cleaning practices is to drink hot water upon getting up in the morning. This ensures proper evacuation as well as it cleans the urinary tract. Half-yearly inner cleaning practices (panchakarma) for cleansing the total body are recommended. These cleaning methods bring equilibrium of the doshas and rejuvenate the body. Before these cleaning practices, the body is subjected to oil massages, hot treatments, sweating and drinking fat, etc. These are also cleansing methods and they also help the body relax through the application of unction and fat. They are helpful for loosening and releasing the dirt from the body. Panchakarma is recommended after the two major seasons, the summer and the winter. For example, in the Northern Hemisphere, it is around March–April and September–October.

Purification of the mind is equally important for good health. A mental state of *santosha* or contentment is a key to good health. Tamasic thoughts like anger, jealousy, competition, excessive attachment, excessive sensual involvement, fear, anxiety, worry, and so on lead to a state of dissatisfaction. Dissatisfaction or *asantosha* gives rise to numerous ailments. A state of *santosha* and a happy disposition is equally essential for health as balanced nutrition, living according to time and place and outer and inner purification. One should make every effort to have sattvic thoughts like compassion, goodness, love and satisfaction, and should try to keep a happy disposition. Tamasic thoughts do not lead to happiness and they enhance *asantosha* (dissatisfaction) and frustration. Therefore, one should make a conscious effort to get rid of the tamasic thoughts. This is done by being aware of them and then through meditative methods make a conscious effort to replace them with sattvic thoughts of peace, harmony and santosha. Just as the outer and inner purification practices are to rejuvenate the body, similarly, the purification of mind promotes mental strength and memory.

It is interesting that Charaka has classified the natural urges into two categories: suppressible and non-suppressible. The non-suppressible urges are those which should not be suppressed as when suppressed they cause various kinds of ailments. These are: urge to urine, faeces, semen, flatus, vomiting, sneezing, eructation, yawning, hunger, thirst, tears, sleep and breathing fast after exertion. The suppressible urges are urge to evil ventures relating to thought, speech and action; urge of greed, grief, fear, anger, vanity, envy and excessive attachment. When one suppresses these urges, one gets the time to think and refrain from these evil thoughts and deeds. This leads us to peace and harmony.

In brief, I would say that the fundamentals of Ayurveda are based upon the principle that nature is a well organised whole where everything has a definite goal and nothing happens without reason or arbitrarily. We human beings are a part of this big and dynamic whole and the same cosmic principles apply to us. We should make every effort to be in harmony with the cosmic rhythm. If we divert too much from the cosmic system, we get out of tune from the universal orchestra. Disharmony and imbalance cause various ailments and mental sufferings. We should make every effort to be in tune with the bigger system for attaining good health, peace and longevity.

Chapter 2

Determining Your Constitution or Prakriti

For practicing an Ayurvedic way of life, it is important that you determine your fundamental constitution or prakriti. Normally the confusion in determining prakriti occurs due to our present state of health. When I describe various kinds of prakriti in my classes, some students are certain about themselves whereas there are others who get very confused and say that they think they have dominance of 'all three' doshas. Many times, the confusion occurs because of the vikriti of one or two doshas. For determining your constitution, you should 'scan yourself' over a longer period of time and from diverse dimensions. If you are having specific symptoms of a particular energy, try to ask yourself if they were always there, particularly when you were a child.

In many modern books on Ayurveda, specially written by foreigners, you will find a very simplistic approach to identify one's prakriti by filling some questionnaires. The findings may or may not be correct or confuse the reader utterly. My method given below is a little more difficult, as it is based upon understanding, observation and inference. It is important to understand that finding one's prakriti is not the sole aim. It is learning to observe oneself and making it a habit to correct all the deviations from prakriti. When we divert from our prakriti or fundamental nature, we have to learn to notice it and take immediate measures to restore back to the state of health or prakriti. Ayurveda is the science of life and for scientific methods of healing, correct diagnosis is the fundamental for applying remedies.

I have given below the three basic dimensions for observing a human being in order to identify his or her prakriti. In each case, many different points should be observed. It is quite possible that you may get confused with some of the observations. But observing other related aspects will solve this problem. I will describe more of this later but first, let us observe a human being from the three dimensions given below.

External Appearance

The most basic observation for determining prakriti as well as to know the state of your health is your outward appearance, like eyes, complexion, nature of the skin, quantity and quality of the hair, body structure and other features of an individual's appearance.

Physical Reactions

The second step to determine prakriti is to observe the physical reactions of people to various life situations like their physical reactions to a stress situation, a shocking news, a good news, an exciting news, an emergency, and so on. When under stress or in a bad situation, some may have frequent stool or urination, the others may get constipation, there are still others who may vomit. Some may just sleep or remain dumbfounded. On long-term stress situations like at work, various persons display diverse reactions. Some may get stomach problems or other ailments related to the digestive system. There are others, who may get different kinds of aches. Another type of persons may start sleeping too much and also get a little depressed.

Behaviour

The way people walk, talk, climb up stairs, enter into a room, answer their doorbells or telephones reveal their prakriti. I have talked above about the physical reactions various people have in different life situations. In this category, notice the behavioural aspect of their reactions. When something goes wrong, people react differently. Does a person get angry or keep patient? While narrating something, various persons have different ways. Similarly, while listening to others, people react differently.

This idea of three-dimensional observation is summed up in Figure 4

Figure 4. Three dimensions of observing a human being for determining prakriti.

EXTERNAL APPEARANCE

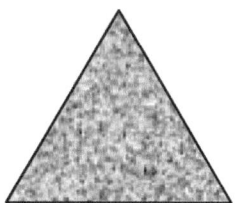

PHYSICAL REACTIONS   **BEHAVIOUR**

Our Internal and External Being

All of us are aware of our external appearance and that is our recognition for ourselves and for the world. To this particular appearance, a name is assigned or rather two names are given. That way, there is clarity about individuals and their identities. What am I externally from my features like shape of my nose, lips, complexion, eyes and other features of the body? I am what I am in comparison to others. When we describe someone's appearance, we generally say things like big eyes, small eyes, sharp nose, small nose, flat nose or upturned nose, and so on. Normally, we observe the external features of others quite spontaneously and naturally. In fact, we observe others more than ourselves as we see ourselves only for that brief time when we are standing in front of the mirror. It is interesting that many people do not know how they look from the side and some are quite surprised to see their side-pose from the photographs. Besides that, when we look at ourselves in the mirror, it is always with indulgence and involvement. Thus, the perception of our outer appearance is vis-à-vis others and also according to the norms of the society.

Prakriti is like the internal appearance of an individual and to learn to perceive that, you have to widen the horizon of your observation and include various aspects of the three dimensions mentioned above. In addition to that, you have to also broaden the sphere of your observation and extend it to other people around you. Expand your mind to look at people not only externally and superficially but also from the

47

point of view of their prakriti. The question is not only about knowing your prakriti, but it is also to observe yourself constantly. Diversion from prakriti to vikriti happens due to various internal and external factors and you have to get used to observing that in order to restore to prakriti. That is the reason that this observation should be like a habit with you and just like you observe yourself or others externally, you need to do the same in reference to prakriti and the related behaviour of the individuals. Thus, the secret of a healthy and long life with strength and vitality is to attend to the state of vikriti immediately and do the needful. For that, you have to train yourself to recognise what I call 'the internal being' of individuals.

Learning to Observe

I will explain below some principal external features and suggest that you observe people around you in reference to these. Get into a habit of looking at the appearance and behaviour of an individual in a different manner than you are used to. Initially, do not do this observation with the idea of determining prakriti. Simply, make an effort to expand your observation.

1. **Hair:**
   a. rough and coarse or soft
   b. thick growth, thin growth or medium

Rough and course hair denote vata, thick growth is for kapha whereas thin growth signifies pitta.

2. **Skin:**
   a. dry
   b. smooth
   c. oily

Dry skin denotes vata, smooth kapha whereas oily skin is a sign for pitta.

3. **Body temperature:**
   a. hot
   b. cold

Hot represents pitta whereas cold is either vata or kapha. Vata is dry and cold whereas kapha is wet and cold.

Body smell:
   a. strong and sometimes bad

    b.   fleshy
    c.   practically none

*Strong body smell denotes pitta whereas fleshy smell is a sign of
kapha. The vata dominant persons who have dry skin have practically
no smell.*

5. **Nails:**
    a.   rough
    b.   bright and pink
    c.   whitish and smooth

*Rough nails are a sign for vata dominance whereas bright and pink
nails are of those who have more fire or pitta. Whitish and smooth
nails are for kapha dominant persons.*

6. **Complexion:**
    a.   radiating
    b.   rather dull
    c.   clear and smooth

*Pitta dominant individuals have a radiating or slightly pinkish com-
plexion whereas a dull complexion denotes vata dominance. Kapha-
dominant persons have clear and smooth complexion.*

7. **Eyes (colour of the retina):**
    a.   clear and white
    b.   greyish and dull
    c.   pink or reddish

*White, dull and reddish represent the domination of kapha, vata and
pitta respectively.*

8. **Body structure and face features:**
    a.   shape of the nose: sharp, fine or thick or in between
    b. shape of the body: delicate or well formed and stable

*The ones with delicate features are pitta dominant whereas slightly
thicker features denote the predominance of kapha. Vata dominating
individuals fall somewhere in between.*

9. **Body movements:**
    a.   fast
    b.   slow and stable
    c.   varied

Kapha-dominant persons are slow and stable whereas fast ones are vata dominant. The dynamic but not excessively fast are pitta dominant individuals.

10. **Way of talking:**
     a. slow and with little gaps
     b. fast
     c. rapid and almost missing some words
     d. dynamic with good self-expression

Slow ones are kapha-dominant, fast ones are pitta-dominant and rapid ones are vata-dominant individuals. Dynamic with good self expression are generally a mixture of pitta and kapha.

11. **Way of listening:**
     a. with patience and attention and slow in grasping
     b. grasping very fast
     c. with impatience and sometimes completing your sentence, attention wandering

Kapha-dominating individual are good listeners whereas vata ones are impatient. Pitta-dominant individuals are quick to grasp.

12. **Climbing up and down the stairs:**
     a. very fast, almost leaving one step in between
     b. very slow and stable
     c. medium
     d. variable

Very fast ones are obviously vata dominating and those who are slow are kapha dominating. Medium or variable are with the predominance of pitta

13. **Response to door bells and telephones:**
     a. very rapid, almost with a jump and making oneself breathless
     b. stable but quite fast
     c. in a rather slow and sluggish manner

The ones who almost jump up with a telephone ring or door bell are predominant in vata and those who let the telephone ring several times before reacting are kapha-dominant. The ones who are stable but fast enough are with pitta-dominance.

14. **Decision making:**
     a. rapid and sometimes rash and impulsive
     b. very slow and sometimes changing one's mind
     c. variable but mostly thoughtful

Kapha-dominant individuals are always slow to decide. Rapid and rather too quick are the vata-dominating persons. Individuals with pitta predominance normally fall in between but are thoughtful in their decisions.

15. Emotional reactions:
   a.   predominant in irritation and worry
   b.   predominant in anger
   c.   generally patient and gulp down emotions

Vata-dominating individuals tend to get irritated and they tend to worry whereas pitta ones have a tendency to get angry rather quickly. Kapha-dominating individuals have patience and tend to suppress their emotions.

Make it a habit to observe the above-mentioned features in persons in the family, at the workplace, amongst your friends or anybody you encounter in day-to-day life. Listen to people carefully when they talk about themselves and pay attention to the following features that will give you an insight into their physiological reactions or other allied features of their personality. From conversations and from the narratives of your colleagues, friends and acquaintances, you may be able to get some information at a slightly profounder level than in the above 15 points, which can be easily observed.

16. Stool:
   a.   immediately after getting up
   b.   after breakfast
   c.   irregular and tendency to have constipation

Pitta-predominant individuals sometimes wake up in the morning because of an urge for stool. Kapha ones tend to have the urge after drinking something or after breakfast. Vata ones have rather irregular stool and have a tendency to get constipated.

17. **Hunger and thirst:**
    a.   eats and drinks a lot
    b.   sometimes a lot, sometimes little
    c.   eats and drinks rather less and in stable quantity

Pitta-dominant individuals have a big appetite and they eat and drink a lot due to the dominance of fire element. Vata-dominating individual vary from one time to the other in their appetite whereas kapha persons eat and drink less.

18. **Sleep:**
    a.   very profound and love to sleep
    b.   needs less sleep and can keep awake easily
    c.   variable and sometimes restless

Kapha-dominating individuals are sleep-loving whereas pitta-dominant persons can do with little sleep. The vata ones are variable and they may get restless sleep at times.

19. **Reaction to weather:**
    a.   dislikes cold weather
    b.   dislikes summer
    c.   dislikes windy weather

Kapha-dominating individuals dislike cold weather, in particular cold and wet. Pitta-dominant individuals suffer easily when it is hot whereas vata ones are very sensitive to windy weather.

Amongst the above 19 points for observation, some are apparent and others are revealed by most people through their conversation. When you learn to observe people a little more than you are used to, you will begin to see another dimension of them. Train your mind for several months in this direction. This observation should be done without thinking of any results or conclusions from it. This is the first step for the formation of a habit to observe.

Interpreting and Inferring the Observations

Once you see that you have become better at observing people around you and yourself as well, try then to interpret all these observations together. You may begin with two or three persons who are closer to you and around you. But you should not ask them any questions. This is a part of your training that you should be able to gather enough observation from external appearances of people and what they reveal about themselves through their conversation.

Any individual observation, if not seen in conjunction with all other related observations and not interpreted in its proper context, may lead to the wrong conclusion. The following examples will help you to sort out your information about determining the prakriti of your chosen cases. Try and choose few cases for your training which are quite different from each other.

Before I begin with different case studies, let me remind you of the following three important points:

- Vata and kapha are cold.
- Pitta is hot.
- The difference between vata and kapha is that vata is dry cold and kapha is wet cold.

Case 1: A person is slow and stable in body movements, lets the telephone ring several times before picking it up and does the same with the door bell. She or he takes always plenty of time to decide. This person has clear and smooth skin, clear eyes and lots of hair. He or she eats and drinks in a limited quantity. Generally, this person loves to sleep and feels tired if the weather is wet and cold. This person has well-connected joints and ligaments. Persons of this category generally postpone things to be done to the next day and that is why their offices and homes are not very well organised.

*This is a clear case of a **kapha** prakriti.*

Case 2: Always complaining of heat, this person sweats a lot and tends to smell bad at times. He/she eats and drinks in plenty but is not fat. Skin is not smooth and gets pimples from time to time but the complexion is bright. Hair growth is not dense. Some of this category may tend to lose hair. This person has plenty of energy. He or she is rather impatient, especially before meals. Persons of this category have a tendency to get easily angry.

*This is a clear case of a **pitta** prakriti.*

Case 3: Speaking and walking rapidly, swift in their actions, these individuals are quick to decide. They are disturbed with windy weather and their complexion is rather dull. Skin gets dried up very quickly and they need to use a lot of oil in dry weather. They get easily irritated and are quick to show emotions like fear, anxiety, etc. They are intolerant to cold and shiver easily. They have usually prominent blood vessels.

*These are the **vata** prakriti persons.*

The Mixed Prakriti

After the three major types of individual constitutions, we turn to other types, which are constituted by the combination of two principal energies. When there is mixed prakriti, an individual may have some traits of both these. This will also be evident from the outward appearance. For example, a thick hair growth (kapha factor) but not a smooth skin as a kapha-dominant person will have. The eyes are not clear white but pinkish. When we come to the personality traits and physical reactions of the persons with mixed prakriti, they have traits of the two types. Let us see some case studies for mixed prakriti.

Case 4: This person is quick to react and decide and is rather rapid in movements. With all these vata characteristic, this person has radiant complexion and has those typical reddish eyes a pitta dominant person will have. This person is very sensitive to food products which are hot in their Ayurvedic qualities like sour and spicy stuff and tends to get pimples or herpes. Some parts of the body are oily like the back and face but arms and legs are dry. Tolerance to heat and cold varies with this person and tends to be angry and impulsive at times.

*This is a person with **vata-pitta** constitution.*

Case 5: With the thick growth of hair and clear skin, well formed body structure, this individual may allude you to be a typical kapha-dominant type but you may feel that he/she is rather rapid in movements and quick to decide. Look very carefully in the eyes of this person with a smoky appearance and that is indicative of the vata aspect of prakriti. It may be a reverse situation where skin and hair may give an appearance of a vata-dominant person but the eyes are clearly indicating the dominance of kapha. This individual may give you an impression of being rather contradictory in her/his nature; at times quiet and tolerant whereas at other times, quite a contrast to that.

*This is an individual with **vata-kapha** constitution.*

Case 6: Here is an individual with fine features and a delicate built but with dense hair growth and clear skin and clear eyes. Or reversing these features, we have an individual with well-formed and strong body, less hair, radiant complexion and slightly reddish eyes. You will notice that the individual of this category can be very tolerant but at times or when provoked, they may explode like a volcano. This person may have phases of eating and drinking a lot, and in contrast to that, may consume very little food and drinks. Imagine that you have known someone who ate a lot when you invited her/him over and six months later, this individual may eat half the quantity when you had specifically made big portions for this person. Over-dressed in winter sometimes, this individual may be enjoying the cold weather at other times.

This is an individual with **pitta-kapha** *prakriti.*

Case 7: Here is an individual who can adjust to most situations and generally gives an appearance of being well balanced and contented. Also in odd and difficult situations, this individual is able to maintain equilibrium. The skin is smooth like that of a kapha person but has also the radiance of pitta. Rapidity of vata is balanced with the stability of kapha. This individual's body is capable of maintaining equilibrium in diverse weather conditions and other external circumstances. Thus, this individual has good stamina and immunity.

This person has **samadosha prakriti** *(equilibrium of all the three energies).*

Are there only seven types of individuals?

It is relatively easy to understand and to be able to determine the prakriti of people or of your own as far as you limit yourself to seven types. However, there are many other factors essential to the seven major types of prakriti, and you will realise that with these variations in each of the above types, we will arrive at a countless number of potential prakriti. But if you have learnt the first major step and have developed the ability to determine the seven major types as distinct from each other, the rest will be easier for you. We will now examine the factors that provide further diversity.

1. **Fundamental energy or** *ojas***:** There are variations of the fundamental vitality, stamina and immunity from one person to another. Let us take an example of ten persons of samadosha prakriti. All of them may show differences despite being in harmony.

They may be different in their fundamental energy levels. Think of that in finer details and imagine them at a scale of from 0.1 to 10. Thus, you have one hundred factors in samadosha. We can apply the same to other six types and we already have numerous types of individuals. To understand this in a more concrete sense, think of the three energies in the form of blocks. In one of the samadosha prakriti person, one block of each energy is present. It could be possible that in another samadosha person, two blocks of each of the energies (vata, pitta and kapha) are present. Like this, let us imagine that there are individuals with up to 10 blocks of each energy. The person with 10 blocks of energy will have the highest of ojas (immunity and vitality). Thus, the fundamental energy quantitatively varies in different human beings.

2. **Degree of dominance:** In the above cases, there are several features to denote the dominance of a particular dosha. It is quite possible that an individual may not have all these characteristics but only some of them. It is also possible that some of these characteristics may be more prominent than the others. All these denote the degree of dominance of that particular vital energy. For example, you know a person who worries a lot. Start noticing the other features described for vata and you will realise that you will find several of these features quite evident in this person. On the other hand, there can be a person who 'tends to worry' and the other allied features may be there to a lesser degree. Thus, there are variations in the degree of dominance of a particular dosha from one individual to another.

3. **Different proportions in mixed prakriti:** There are three types of mixed prakriti but the proportion of each of the two dominant dosha may vary. For example, in a person with vata-pitta prakriti, the two energies may be present in any proportion. If there is more pitta than vata, we can call it a pitta-vata prakriti. Imagine the similar variations in vata-kapha and pitta-kapha types or prakriti.

Just like millions and billions of people on this earth can be distinguished from each other on the basis of their external features, the same is true for their inner being or prakriti. You should consider the prakriti of a person like his or her inner face. Keep in mind the seven major types of prakriti and allow for some variations in them. With practice, your horizon will gradually enhance and you will be able to spontaneously observe people for their prakriti as you now see and distinguish them outwardly.

Some Interesting Experiences with Prakriti

My experiences in Ayurveda seminars in Europe may be useful to state here as they might help you clarify some doubts that may arise after having read the above description.

Ayurveda has become very popular during the last decade particularly in German-speaking countries. There are some schools which have sprung up to provide some training for a month or two and then these 'graduates' teach or even practise. Evidently, these 'teachers' or 'practitioners' acquire very superficial knowledge of the subject. We in India say that one need several lives to learn the wisdom of Ayurveda. One of the beliefs of some such schools is to glorify certain types of prakriti and to condemn the other types. This wrong notion is further propagated when other people learn that from teachers trained with this notion.

A young lady who is teaching Ayurveda and yoga in Germany invited me to do a one-week seminar with her and her students. She herself was convinced that pitta is the best prakriti and that is why she is a brilliant and a charming person. Kapha prakriti was downgraded in her opinion and she thought these people were slow and are a drag and perhaps also not so intelligent. In this seminar, I told her that she had a pitta-kapha prakriti and that was almost unacceptable for her. It took me several days to completely convince her of the rational basis the kapha features predominant in her body and personality. This poor lady was quite unaware that the great Albert Einstein also had pitta-kapha prakriti.

Variations in the universe do not mean that certain things are good or bad. There are varied colours, smells, vegetations, seasons, and so on. We should look at the prakriti or the individual constitution in a similar manner. The great factor in a creative genius is not what prakriti he or she has. It is the fundamental energy that plays a great role. Each type of prakriti amongst the seven fundamental types has its own specific characteristics. The same basic quality can be used for a positive or negative purpose. For example, dominance of fire element can be used for creative purpose or it can find its outlet in the form of anger. Air and ether elements may be used to expand oneself in terms of experience and wisdom or to acquire a thoughtless rapidity that ultimately turns out to be negative. Stability of the water and earth elements can be used to solve the intricate problems or it can be just wasted by diminishing one's mobility or being lazy.

In a seminar elsewhere in Germany, the organiser was convinced that kapha prakriti was the best and that people with this prakriti were blessed with longevity. In another seminar, when I gave examples of different types of prakriti from amongst the students, one young lady started crying and said that I should not have revealed that before everybody. Many a times in such situations, people took prakriti as some kind of ailment or initial symptoms of an ailment. This attitude has now changed over the years with a constant spread of Ayurveda.

A friend of mine in Germany is ready to accept anything that is based on rationality and has some scientific basis. He was rather conservative in his view of the medicine and science that came from the orient but was extremely impressed when I told him about his prakriti and various physical and personality factors based upon that. What impressed him the most was the inter-link between various aspects of his character related to the element fire; to name a few—his reddish complexion, his anger, his brilliance and his resistance to cold.

In a weekend seminar, after I devote half a day on the theme of prakriti with examples and so on, there are always persons who come to me and tell me a story about their prakriti. Generally it is that they got themselves 'diagnosed' from someone or through questionnaires from a book but they were not convinced with that diagnosis.

It is better not to know your prakriti than to have a wrong idea about yourself. It is more reliable to try and do your own analysis with your own wisdom or seek the help of an appropriate Ayurvedic physician than to consult a person with little knowledge. It is not all that difficult to learn to analyse prakriti and in your own case it is the easiest. I have summarised below in Figure 5 the steps we have gone through to acquire the knowledge about prakriti.

Figure 5. Steps for identifying your prakriti

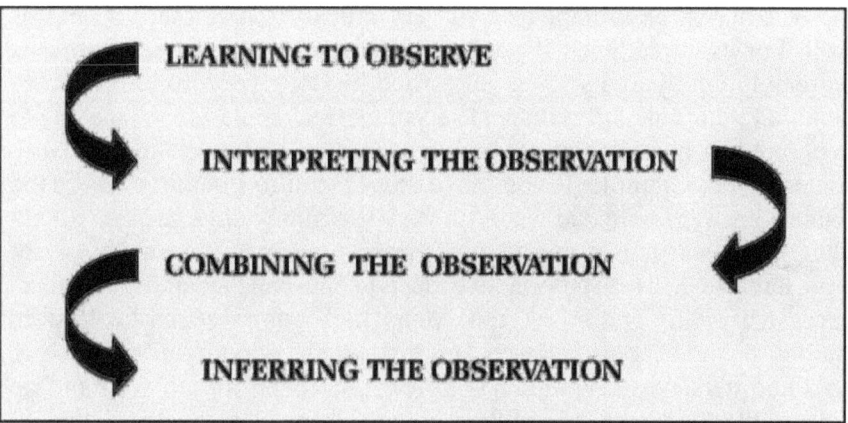

Prakriti—A Self Organising System

It is important to learn that the bodily system has its perfect organisation and if this system is affected or attacked by external forces, it makes an effort on its own to reorganise and stabilise itself. The system makes every effort to revert back to its original nature. For example, if we get a small cut on the finger, it heals after some time. If we eat some bad food, the body throws it out in one way or another. If we feel cold, our body shivers to warm itself up. If it is hot, we sweat and the body cools down.

It is easy to understand this concept if you observe nature. The cosmos and the body are made of the same five fundamental elements. The body has an autonomous organisation which is similar to the cosmic organisation. When there are disturbances in nature due to too much rain, drought, storm, cyclones, excessive heat or cold, earthquake and so on, after a while, nature organises itself back to normality.

Deviation from prakriti to vikriti

You have already learnt that deviation from prakriti is vikriti or a state of non-health. Non-health does not necessarily mean a feeling of being unwell or ill, it could be just a state where one does not have one's optimum energy level. It is important to understand that you are likely to get a vikriti of your dominating dosha or doshas from factors such as weather, unbalanced nutrition, change of place, overwork, too much travelling or emotional factors, etc. A behaviour that is not corresponding to external environments will very quickly vitiate other doshas as well. For example, even if your prakriti is not vata but the weather is extremely windy and you eat cold food or sleep very little, it is probable that your vata will vitiate. The same effect could take place due to geographical change and not living according to that change of environment. For example, if you move from Delhi to Frankfurt where the winters are very cold and wet with very few sunny days and you do not alter your food habits and way of living, you may get kapha vikriti. You have to learn to stay active despite the weather and not eat an excessively fatty and sweet diet. Many Indian immigrants to Western Europe or other cold countries stay too much indoors due to the wet, cold and dark weather. One has to learn to cover oneself well and go out despite the weather. Similarly, people from cold countries stay too much in the sun when they are in locations with sun shine. There is an amusing old Indian saying to this effect: 'Only dogs and Englishmen go out on a summer afternoon'.

Everything in this universe is fluid and not rigid and so are our physical and mental reactions to the environment. The change from prakriti to vikriti will keep happening due to diverse factors. The role of Ayurvedic practice is to diagnose oneself with simple observations of the urine, stool, taste in the mouth, complexion, etc., and then take immediate action to help the body re-establish its prakriti.

The body itself is capable of reverting back from vikriti to prakriti. For example, if we eat too many pitta-promoting things and get too much heat in the body, mild diarrhoea may occur to throw out the excessive heat from the body. If we consume something that is hard to digest or is spoilt, our body throws it out to regain its balance. In such cases, you should not take any medication to hinder the process of nature and let the events take their own course. The body has a perfect system and our intervention should be to help nature. Charaka gives an example of a fallen man who will get up anyway but if someone gives him a hand, it will be easier for him. Similarly, in case of a diversion from prakriti, we should help the process of recovery by taking appropriate measures like balanced food, rest, massage, baths and other such simple measures. Due to an external attack of bacteria or viruses or due to an injury, prakriti deviates to vikriti. In such cases, first of all appropriate medication and a proper diet are required for healing and then the body gradually comes back to its natural state.

A daily diagnosis of your state of health is described in the next chapter. Later in the last chapter of the book, various home remedies are given to help change vikriti to prakriti. You may proceed in the following manner:

1. Determine your prakriti as has been described above.

2. Diagnose daily your state of health with the diagnostic methods described in the Morning Programme (next chapter).

3. If you find any diversion from prakriti to vikriti, take different measures with your diet and medications as has been described in the last chapter of the book.

If you are recovering from some illness or injury, make every effort to revert to prakriti and enhance your ojas as described in the last chapter of the book.

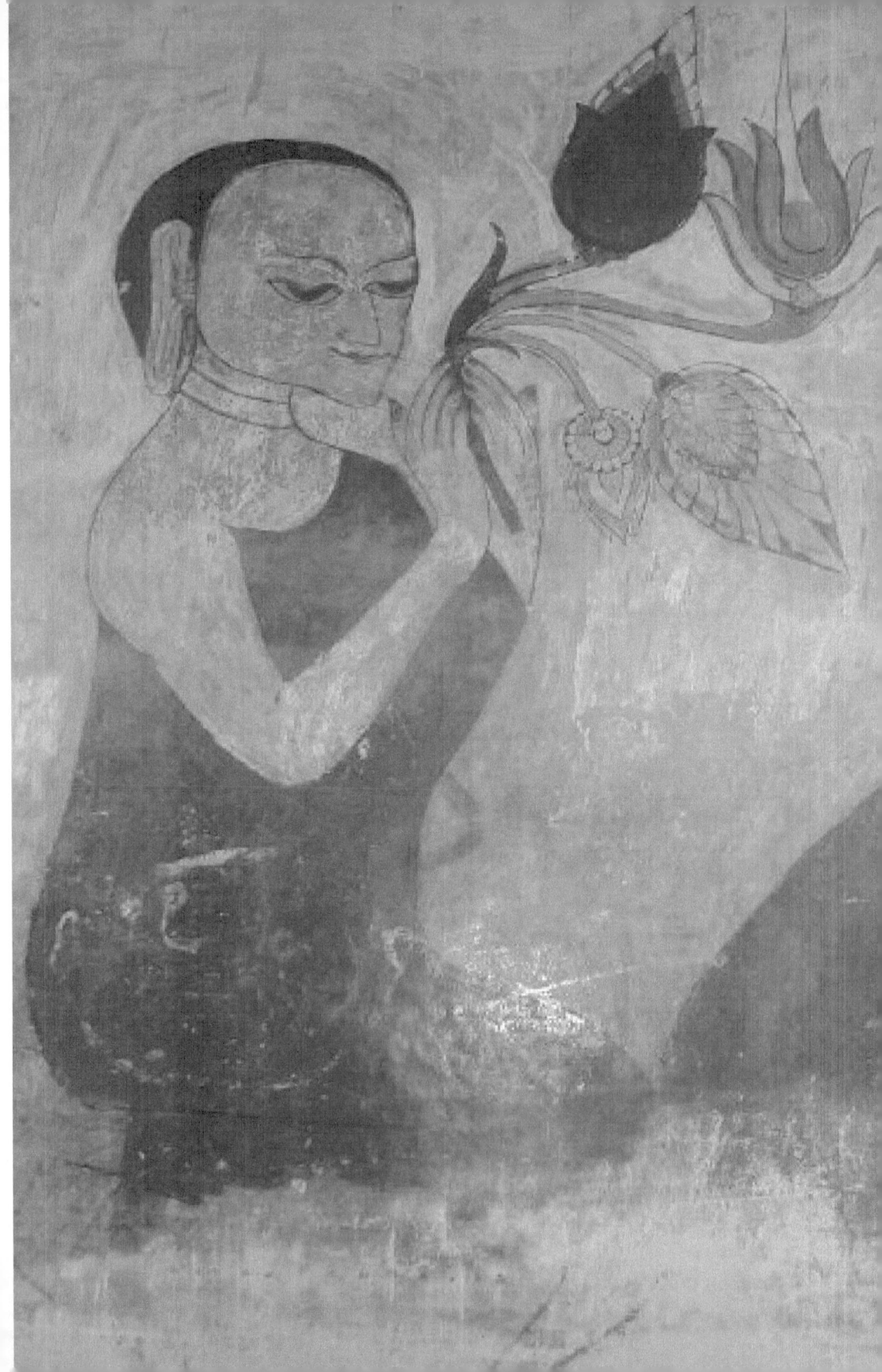

Chapter 3

Dincharya—The Daily Routine

PRATAHCHARYA—THE MORNING PROGRAMME

The morning programme includes various activities to awaken our consciousness towards our surroundings, invoke the cosmic energy and bring peace of mind and physical strength. The following practices will help you do your daily diagnosis and to determine if you have any vikriti. They help purify and rejuvenate both body and mind and help you to begin your day with sattva or stillness. Sattva enhances your work-efficiency and creativity. It also gives you radiance. The Ayurvedic bath has also a spiritual dimension; it not only cleans the body and vitalises the *srotas* or the energy channels but also purifies the mind and helps heal ailments.

Mental and physical purification

Upon getting up in the morning...

Wake up gradually and think of the sun that brings the morning for you. Morning means another day of life.

Sit down and turn your face towards the east, think of the sun and visualise its image in your mind. Repeat the following in your mind:

O Sun! I am grateful to you for another day of life. Bless me so that I see many more days like this. May my five senses work until the end of my life! Bless me so that I live a long and healthy life. I am grateful to you for another day of life. Guide me with your light, show me the right way so that I always take right decisions. Protect me and bless me with the feeling of well-being. I am grateful to you for another day of life. I am grateful to you for another day of life. I am grateful to you for another day of life.

Pranayama

Pranayama is a technical term for various breathing practices described in yoga. Breathing is our link with the cosmos. It is the demonstration of being alive. More details of pranayama are given in the box below.

After the above mantra for the sun, take five deep breaths in the following manner. This practice requires two minutes.

1. Inhale gradually and smoothly and take all the prana energy to the region of your solar plexus. Hold the breath there while you concentrate upon this region. Exhale gradually and smoothly and when all the air is out, do not inhale for a moment and keep your lungs without air. Concentrate on your solar plexus.
2. For the second breath, inhale in the same slow and gradual manner and send the prana energy to your navel region. Hold the breath while you concentrate on the navel region and then let it out gradually and smoothly. Continue to concentrate on the navel region and hold the lungs without air.
3. With the third breath send your prana energy between your navel and your feet while you inhale. Hold the breath inside and let the prana circulate in the lower back and legs. Exhale gradually while your concentration is steady on the lower region and then hold the lungs without air for a moment.
4. Your fourth breath should take the prana energy to your head region, let it stay there while you hold the breath and then exhale smoothly and gradually. Continue concentrating on the head region while you hold the lungs without air.
5. The fifth breathing practice is a little more complicated than the previous ones as it involves sending the prana energy to your whole body. While you inhale gradually and smoothly, circulate your prana energy in your whole body. The technique involves taking the prana energy once to your head and then through shoulders and neck to your hands and then through the thorax and abdomen to your legs and feet. Hold the breath and think of your entire body. Gradually exhale in a slow and smooth manner while concentrating on your entire body. Hold the lungs without air for a moment.

PRANAYAMA

For doing the above breathing practices in a proper and efficient manner, it is essential to understand pranayama.

The literal meaning of pranayama is the control over one's prana. Prana means life itself or consciousness. The cause of consciousness is soul in the body but the factor that holds body and soul together and is responsible for a continuous vivacity is prana (breathing). When prana stops, the body is separated from the soul and eventually dies. Prana or the continuous cosmic energy comes to us through our breathing process. Thus, breathing is not simply a mechanical phenomenon that gives fuel in the form of oxygen for making the body-machine work as is thought by those who compare the living body to a machine. The phenomenon of breathing is our link with the cosmos and in the form of air we inhale cosmic energy and not merely the required oxygen.

A large part of the air consists of nitrogen which also makes up a substantial part of our body in the form of proteins. There are many other elements of earth (carbon, silicon, calcium, phosphorus, etc.) in the air. Since we have all the fundamental elements in the atmosphere which we breathe in, the related subtle elements are obviously also taken in. The vital quality of the air changes with place, time of the day, weather, climate, etc., and that affects our lives directly. We must remember that the intake of vital air is a phenomenon that is linked with our whole life—it is life itself and that is why the sages called it prana.

Initiation into Pranayama

Step 1: First you sit down cross-legged or in lotus posture. Make sure that your backbone is straight and your body is completely relaxed. Begin to inhale in a regular but gradual manner almost to your total capacity, fully concentrate on the prana, its rhythm and follow its journey inside you. Let yourself loose from the effort of inhaling and stay still while the prana is inside you. Keep it in as long as you can

65

and then exhale gradually with the same rhythm. Do not let your concentration divert from your breath. When you have exhaled completely, stay without air a little an concentrate on your inner space. Repeat this whole process several times and gradually increase the time you inhale and exhale as well as holding with air and without air. Inhalation and exhalation should be of equal length and the pauses in between about half as long. This gives a general idea of the technique; there is no need to look at a watch.

Step 2: After the initial practice in Step 1, energise separately the left and right side of the body with prana. These
two sides represent tamas and rajas in the body respectively. They can also be compared to moon (left) and sun (right). This practice is done by closing one nostril and breathing exclusively through the other. Pick up your left hand and close your left nostril with your thumb and inhale through your right nostril **(Figure 6)**. Then hold the air inside by closing also your right nostril with your ring finger **(Figure 7).** Now lift your ring finger and exhale through the right side and replace the ring finger again to hold the lungs without air. Repeat the procedure six to ten times exclusively with right nostril. Make sure that your left nostril is kept closed properly. Repeat the same with the left nostril while you keep your right nostril closed.

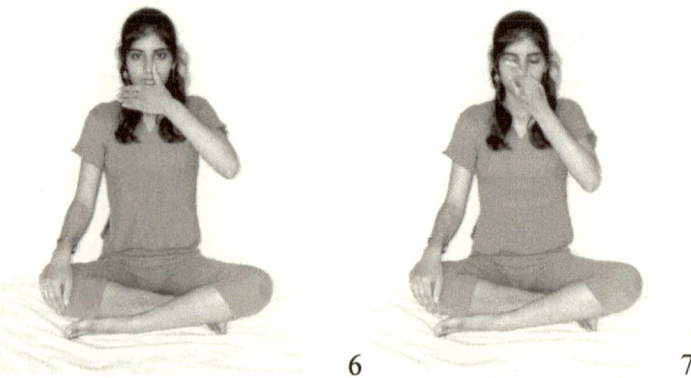

6 7

Step 3: Inhale through the right nostril first while the left is kept closed with your thumb. Then close the right nostril also with your ring finger to hold the air inside. Let the air out from the left nostril by lifting the thumb and continue to keep the ring finger on the right nostril. Close also the left nostril now to keep the lungs without air.

Inhale through the left nostril and continue the procedure. In other words, you inhale through one nostril and exhale though the other, and for the next round, you inhale through the nostril from which you have previously exhaled. Repeat this also six to ten times.

Step 4: Finally, you inhale through both the nostrils but close them with your thumb and ring finger when you have inhaled and when you are holding the lungs without air.

After Getting Up...

We cannot look inside our body. Urine and stool bring us some information about the inner activities and the state of the body. They are the remnants that body has thrown out as *mala* or excrement and they are the result of many actions and reactions in the body. A healthy body is a perfect system and it shows when something is wrong. Thus, urine and stool diagnosis provides us with an easy daily check on ourselves and helps us to keep the bodily organisation in a perfect shape.

Urine and its diagnosis

When you go to relieve yourself, observe the colour and quality of your urine and diagnose it to find out your state of health. Following are different diagnosis of urine:

- The healthy urine should be transparent and nearly like water.
- Turbid urine speaks for excess of air element in your body (vata).
- Yellow urine is indicative of too much heat in your body (pitta).
- If your urine has foam, it is because of the disturbance of water and earth element (kapha) in your body.

Stool and its diagnosis

According to your prakriti, some of you may have evacuation immediately after getting up (pitta) whereas others may have a little after getting up and moving around (kapha). There are still others who may have urge for stool after drinking hot water (vata). Observe your stool carefully and know about your state of health. Following are different diagnosis of stool.

- The healthy stool should be neither too hard and nor too soft in consistency and should be well formed.

- Dry and dark coloured stool in the shape of small balls speaks for vata vikriti.

- Stool of watery consistency and greenish colour denotes pitta vikriti.
- Sticky and whitish stool shows kapha vikriti.

Washing the eyes

After having relieved yourself, wash your eyes and rinse your mouth. Splash your eyes with cold water. Throw water with force on your open eyes. Repeat it 5–6 times. This practice rejuvenates the eyes and the vision.

Cleaning the mouth and the tongue

While cleaning your teeth, concentrate entirely on them and clean them properly and tenderly preferably with an Ayurvedic toothpaste or tooth powder. Rinse your mouth and clean your tongue. Stick it out and either clean it with the tongue cleaner or with a soft tooth brush (Figures 8-9). Your throat will make a sound during this process and will also exercise your stomach.

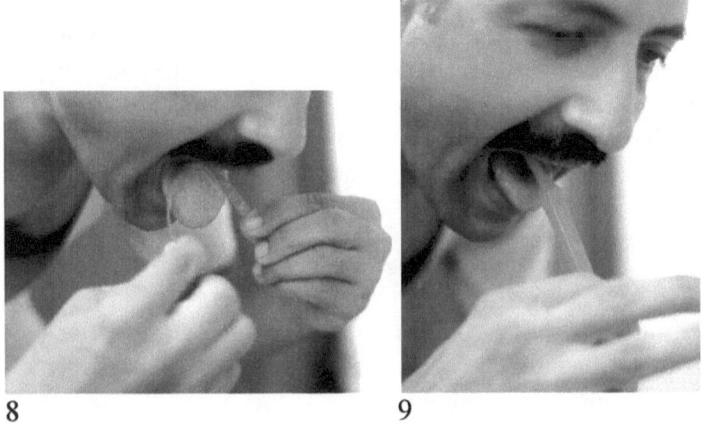

8   9

Drinking hot water

Drink a glass of hot water (about 250 ml.). Let the water stand overnight and heat it up before you drink it. Preferably, drinking water should be prepared by cooking it with some cardamom as described below. Cardamom water can be stored for a few days.

In case you suffer from constipation or partial evacuation, the quantity of water should be increased to two glasses.

CARDAMOM WATER

Put 2 to 3 litres of potable water in a pot. Crush 3-4 cardamom after taking off their pods and add these in water. Boil the water for about 3 minutes. In case there is any danger of biological contamination, boil the water for about 15 minutes. Water should be boiled on low fire and with the lid on. Let the water cool down and store it in bottles. For your morning drinking water, take the required quantity from this and heat it up before drinking. This water may be taken any time during the day to quench the thirst. Cardamom water quenches thirst better than the ordinary water.

Cardamom is good for throat, voice, digestion and heart. It is a balanced spice and helps bring the equilibrium of three doshas.

Exercise, yoga or a walk

Do not lie down after drinking hot water. The best is to do some yogic exercises. Those of you who have already learnt yogic exercises and asanas (postures), I suggest doing Surya Namaskar (Prostration to the sun) 12 times. It has 12 different postures and takes about 12 minutes to do 12 times. However, you may do only 3 or 5 or 7 times. Surya Namaskar (SN) will give you energy for the day.

For those who are rather short of time or are beginners in yoga, I have developed some alternative exercises derived from yoga which require only about five minutes and I call these '**The Five Element Energy Programme (FEEP)**'.

If you feel that you do not have enough energy to do yogic exercise or are suffering from weakness and fatigue due to some ailment or you lack energy due to age, then the alternative is to have a 5 to 10 minutes walk in the fresh air. In any case, you have three options and the details of FEEP and SN are given below.

Five Element Energy Programme (FEEP)

This programme involves a total of 7 different exercises and they are devoted to the five fundamental elements that constitute us.

Rocking movements for the element wind

Lie down on your back. Bend your legs and bring them to your chest. Put both your arms around your bent legs and clasp your hands together. Lift your head up towards your knees and rock your body forward and backward seven times (Figure 10). Think of the element wind during this time. It is the element wind that circulates blood in your body and makes you walk, talk, think and excrete. It is this element that moves your food into your alimentary canal. In the second part of this exercise, make the same posture initially, but roll the body sideways seven times (Figure 11)

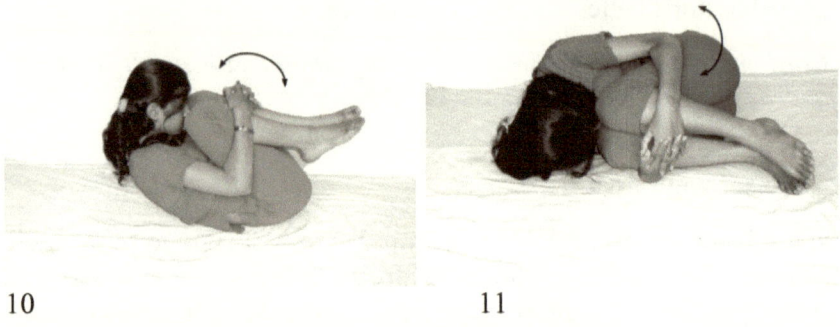

10   11

Whole body stretching for the element ether

Lie down on your back and stretch your arms upwards so that your body occupies the maximum space. Keep your arms straight and parallel to each other. Think of the bright and blue limitless sky and stay in this posture for five breaths (Figure 12). Gradually raise yourself from the waist without moving your legs and with your head parallel to your arms (Figure13). Bend forwards very slowly and smoothly and touch your feet with your hands (Figure 14). In this bent down position, think of the sky full of stars on a dark night. Your stretched out body gradually folds and occupies half the space in this exercise just as the sky seems to be shrunken at night due to darkness.

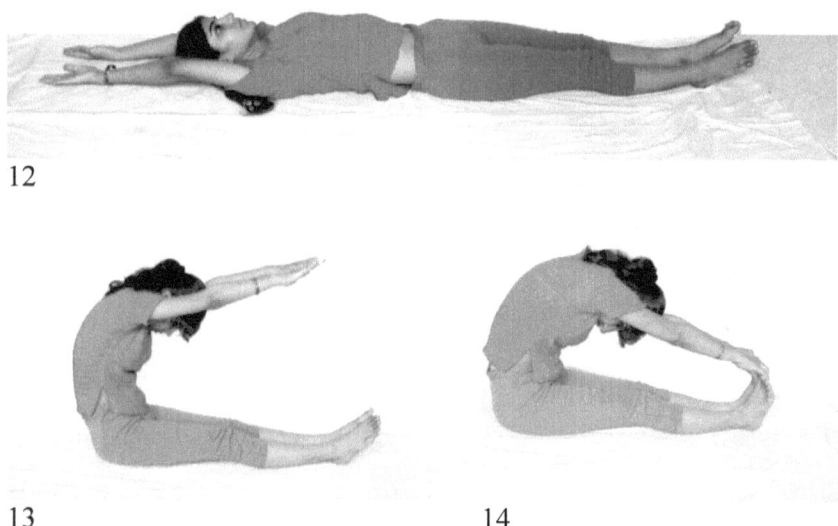

12

13   14

Three standing exercises for the element fire

A. Stand straight with your feet a little apart and palms together. Your body weight should be resting equally on both feet (Figure15). Let yourself loose and take your torso slightly backwards so that your backbone is straightened. Stay like this for five deep breaths and concentrate on the sun.

B. Stretch your hands upwards and bend backwards in this position (Figure16). Straighten yourself and unfold your hands. Bend forward with the stretched arms and touch your feet with your hands while thinking of various colours of fire (Figure 17).

C. Stand straight and bend your knees in such a manner as if you were going to sit (Figure 18). Keep your back straight. Concentrate on your solar plexus and think of the fire which is inside you and which provides you warmth. Make this posture for three breaths.

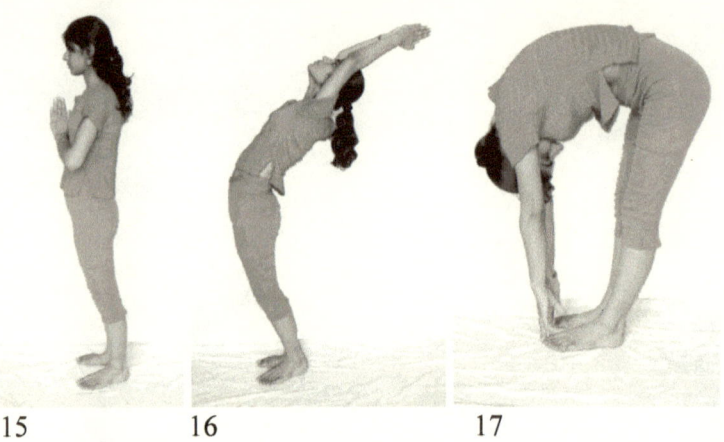

15   16   17

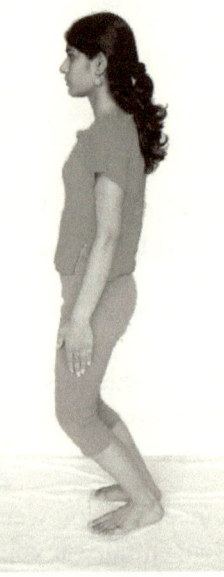

Standing on the Knees and Swinging for the Element Water

Stand on your knees and put your left leg forward to make a posture as shown in Figure 19. At this stage, your weight is largely on the right knee; your right arm is parallel to your right thigh. Put your left hand on your left knee. Swing your body (from the torso) back and forth for five times and think of the flowing water (Figure 20-21). Repeat the same with the right leg forward and while swinging your body five times, think of the blood flowing in your body, which is flowing like rivers in nature.

18

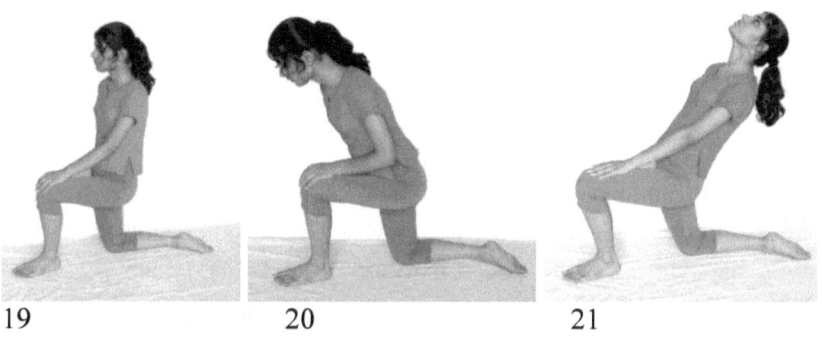

19   20   21

Sitting on the heals for the element earth

After the above exercise, come back to the posture of standing on your knees and then sit on your heals. Put your hands on your knees and let yourself loose (Figure 22). Sit like this for five deep breaths and think of the element earth that provides us food and shelter. Take your hand behind your back, clasp them and bend your head forward to touch the floor (Figure 23). Wish for the stability of the earth element in your body that provides you the structure. Also wish for the equilibrium of all the five elements in your body.

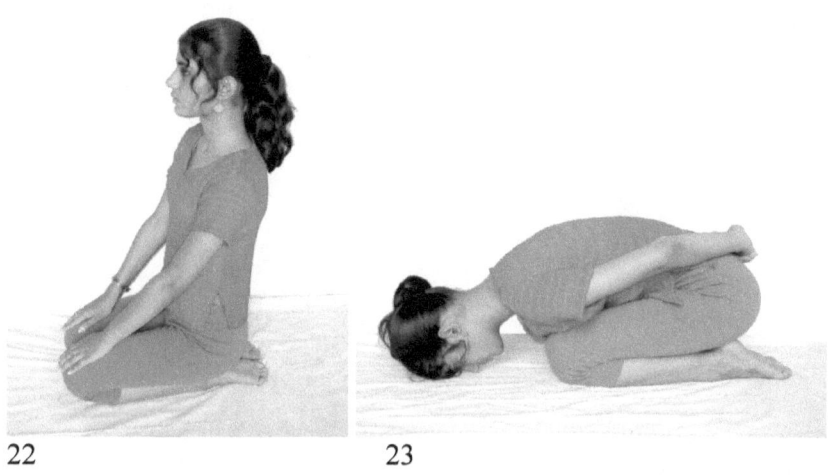

22   23

Surya Namaskar or Prostration to the Sun

Surya Namaskar (SN) involves making 12 different postures one after the other. Either learn the postures one by one gradually or learn with a teacher.

1. Face the direction of the sun and stand with palms facing each other. Your legs should be about 20 cm apart from each other. Put your torso slightly backward and let yourself loose (Figure 24). Close your eyes and concentrate on the image of the sun. You may repeat the Gayatri mantra or another simple mantra for the sun like, *Om suryaye namah.* Repeat this mantra 5 or 7 or 11 times.

2. Slowly raise your hands upwards until your head is between your two arms and bend backward in this position (Figure 25). Lean as far back as you comfort-ably can, making sure that your head is always between your arms.

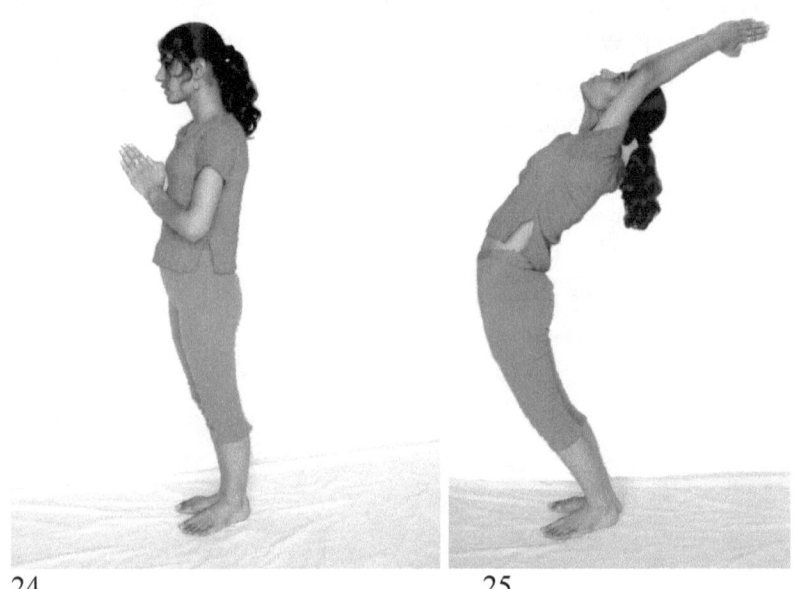

24   25

3. Straighten your body gradually, take your hands apart from each other and make your arms straight, with both palms facing forward. Bend forward and then downward and touch the ground with your hands on both sides of your feet (Figure 26). Your legs should be straight in this posture and knees should not bend. If your body is not flexible enough to touch the ground, do not force yourself. With repeated practice, you will be able to become flexible.

4. From the above posture, shift your weight to your hands and your left leg and stretch the right leg backwards so that it rests on the knee and the front part of your foot. In this process, your left leg is folded. Bend your head backward (Figure 27).

5. Bring your bent head forward and shift your body weight to both your hands. Stretch back the right leg. Make a straight line with your body by shifting your weight to your hands and toes. Your head should be in line with the rest of your body (Figure 28).

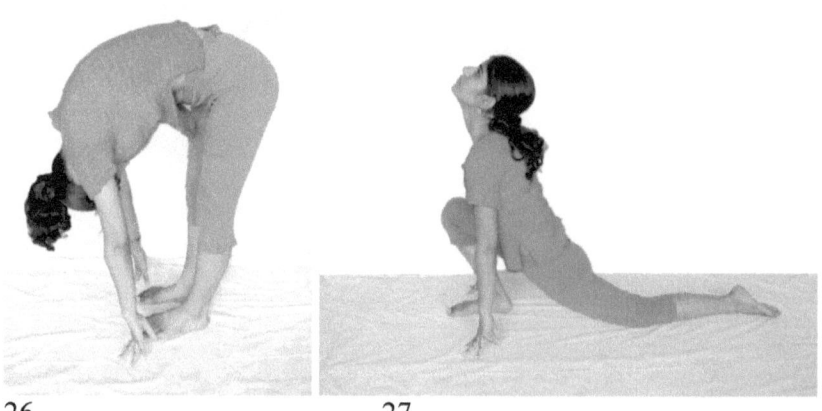

26   27

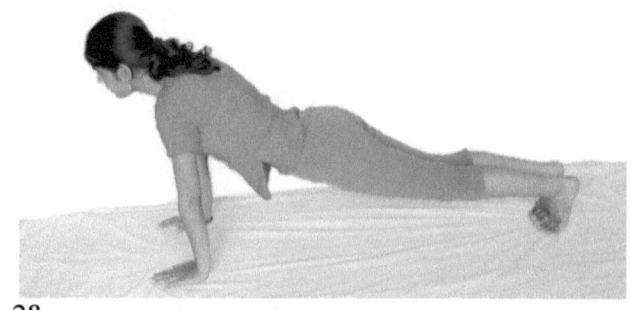

28

6. In position 5, you are touching the ground with four parts of your body. This position is made by touching the ground with eight parts of the body and that is why it is called *ashatanaga pranama* (prostration with eight parts of the body). In addition to your hands and feet, touch the ground with both your knees, your chest and forehead (Figure 29). Your stomach and thighs should not touch the ground.

7. Put your weight on hands and feet and gradually raise your head. Bend your head backward as far as you comfortably can (Figure 30).

8. Slowly lower your head from the previous position, raise your body in the middle while putting your weight on your hands and feet. Your head should remain between your arms, whereas your feet should be in a flat position with the soles touching the ground (Figure 31).

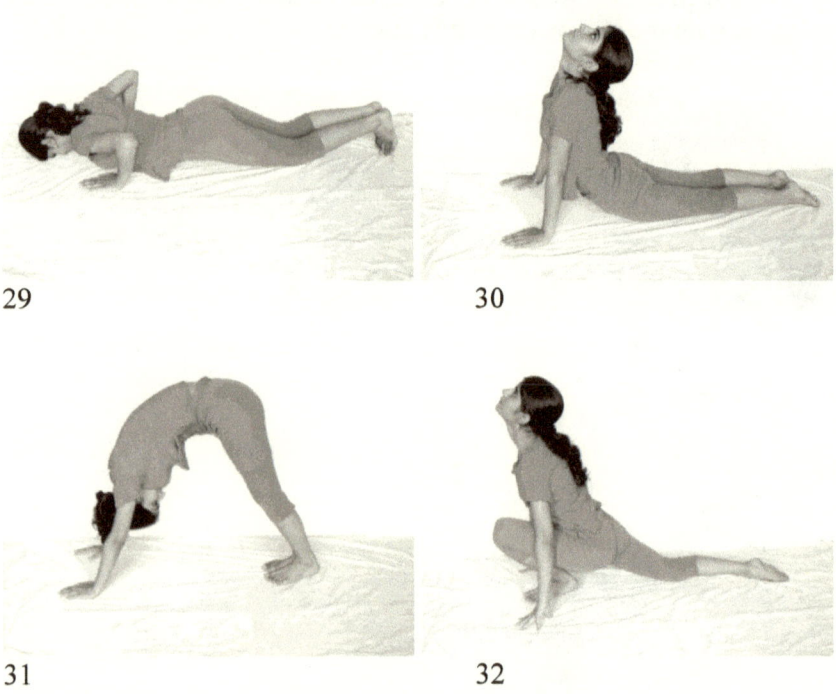

29

30

31

32

9. Bring the right leg forward, stretch back the left leg, put your weight on your hands and make your arms straight. Bend your head backward. This position is the same as position 4 except that here the right leg is forward instead of the left leg (Figure 32).

10. This position is the same as Position 3. From position 9, bring your stretched leg forward and put this foot parallel to the other foot between your two hands. In this process, your body will be slightly lifted. Keep your legs straight and do not bend your knees (Figure 33). 11. Straighten your body from the previous position and raise your arms upward; join your hands and bend backward as you did in Position 2 (Figure 34).

12. This is the last position and here you come back to Position 1, from where you started (Figure 35).

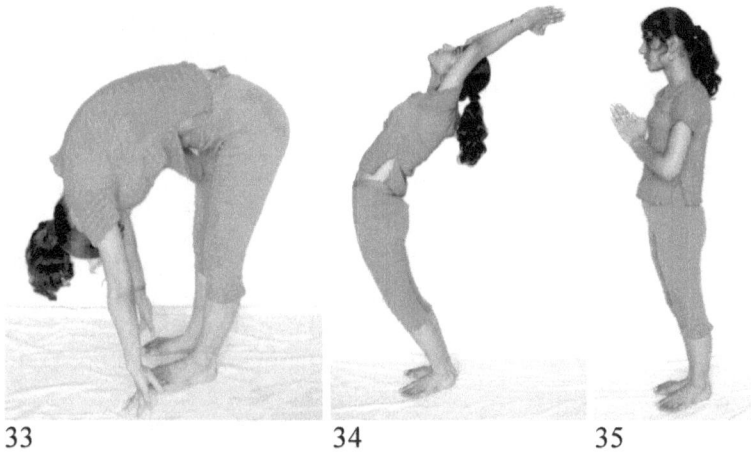

33   34   35

The Ayurvedic bath... or shower

After your exercise, leave a gap of a few minutes before you take a shower or a bath.

Ayurvedic bath is different from the Western concept of taking a bath by sitting in water. It is done by putting water on you from a bucket or a source of water with the help of a small container. A shower can also serve this purpose.

The Ayurvedic bath has various little practices that I have compiled together for the rejuvenation of the body. You require putting water on your body several times. Your mental state is equally important and this bath is meant to clean the body, energise it, purify the mind, throw away bad thoughts and enhance the healing process in case of disorders.

For an Ayurvedic bath, you require:

1. Good soap prepared with oil, so that it does not dry the skin
2. From time to time 200 ml of pure, fresh, untreated milk (raw, not boiled)
3. Coconut oil, olive or sesame oil and mustard oil
4. A massage brush with long handle
5. Medium hot bathing water

Wet your body with water (Figure 36). Rub some soap between your palms and put some sesame oil on the soap in your palms (Figure 37). Mix the soap and the oil by rubbing your palms together (Figure 38). Apply this mixture on your whole body with some force (Figure 39). You may have to repeat this process of mixing soap and oil several times to have enough for your whole body.

Pour water on yourself to wash off the soap and keep rubbing your body with your hands to take out the last traces of soap. Let the water flow on your body and take away the entire dirt. Concentrate your thoughts on your body and wish that all the impurities from your body and mind are washed away. Impurities of mind are jealousy, greed, excessive desire for things, etc. If you have a pain or a disorder, let it go away along with the dirt and perspiration from your body. Let the flowing water take all this away and purify your body and mind.

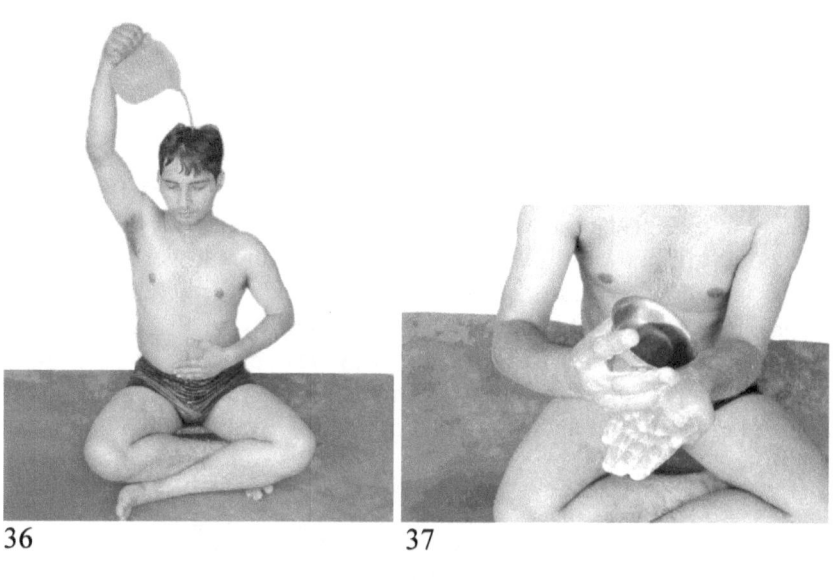

36
37

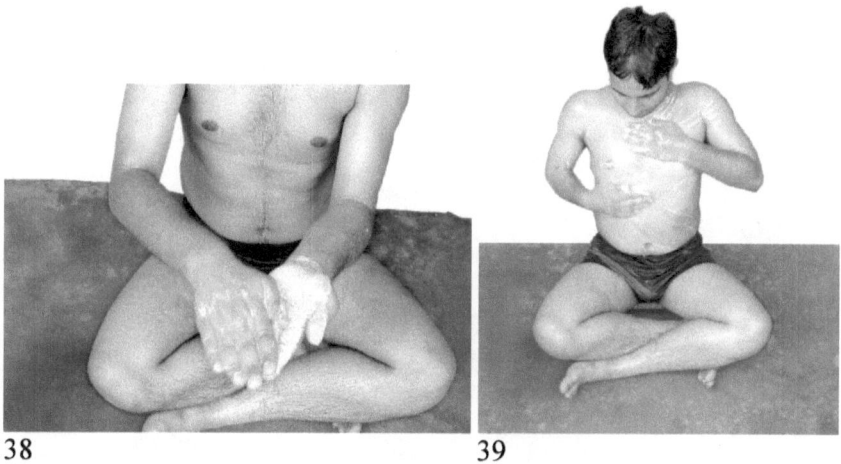

38
39

From time to time, take some milk in a small container and apply it on your body little by little by taking some in your palm (Figure 40). Rub well to clean the body. When you clean your body with milk, you do not need soap. Milk purifies very well. Wash off the milk with water.

After the soap or milk is washed away, massage your whole body with a massage brush. Pay special attention to all the joints and the areas where there is more flesh like the thighs, hips and abdoman (Figure 41). Massage the neck region and the middle of the back (the place of the vertebral column) several times (Figure 42). This massage will activate and rejuvenate your body. Pour hot water on yourself after the massage and apply some warm coconut oil all over your body. Keep the coconut oil bottle in hot water as at temperatures lower than 25^0 C, this oil is solidified. Rub the body properly and everywhere with oil. Oil provides strength to the body and tranquillity to the mind. After you have rubbed the oil well and the body has absorbed it, pour some warm water on yourself to wash off the extra oil. Wish that your disorders, imbalances and pains might be washed away from your body with this flowing water.

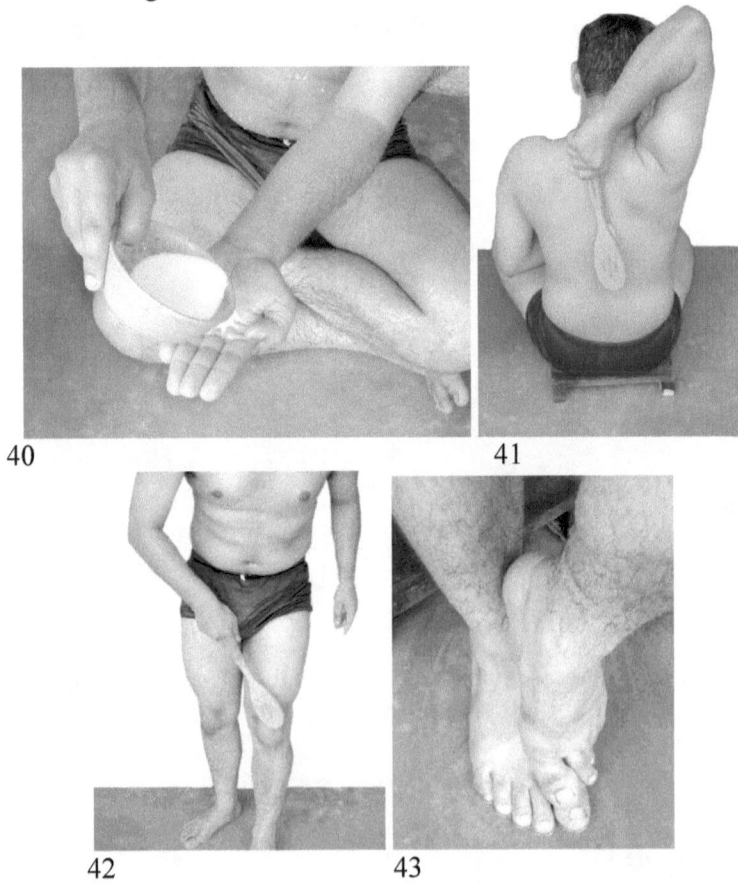

40

41

42

43

Note: Coconut oil is cold in nature and is good to use in summer. But in heated houses, it may be equally used in winter. Sesame and olive oil are hot in their nature but for massage they should be cooked at very high temperatures, if possible, with some herbs. I have given a simple recipe for making a massage oil in Chapter 4. Persons of pitta prakriti can always use coconut oil. For those who have kapha and vata prakriti, it is good to use sesame oil especially in winter. Sesame oil prepared with Ayurvedic ingredients is good for all types of prakriti for strengthening and beautifying the skin.

Massage the toe of your left foot with right foot and the other way around (Figure 43). Similarly, massage your thumbs and press on the space between your thumb and the index finger (Figure 44). Finally, massage your ears by pressing their various parts.

Mustard oil is used to clear the nasal passage at the end of the bath. Dip two fingers in mustard oil, stick them in your nostril and inhale (Figure 45). This will cause sneezing. Then blow your nose strongly. In case you are hesitant to inhale the strong mustard oil, at least blow your nose strongly after the bath. Finish the bath by pouring some hot water on yourself and wishing yourself a peaceful day.

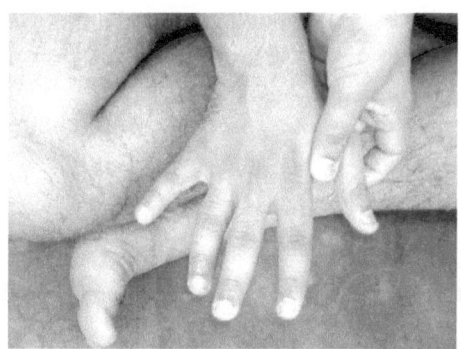 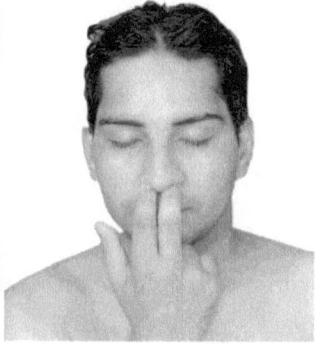

44   45

Morning time thoughts

Morning time is holy, try to speak minimum during the morning hours. Try to silence your mind and keep it free from the thoughts of other persons, events, worries or problems. Concentrate only on the purification of your body. If thoughts about problems or related to your day's activities come to your mind, make a conscious effort to silence your mind by thinking of the sun which has brought you another day of life. At least until your bath, keep such thoughts away.

Things to remember

From the Ayurvedic point of view, do not do the following, as they are injurious to your health:

- Do not jump out of your bed abruptly. Your body and mind need time to alter from the state of inertness (tamas) to activity (rajas). This transition should be brought about softly and tenderly.

- It is observed that some people jump out of their beds and go under a shower, quickly dress up and go to work. Many of these may suffer from constipation, which is the root cause of several ailments. If you do this, you are being nasty to your body and the results of this nastiness will tell upon your health sooner or later.

- Evacuation is a very important part of the morning programme and do not postpone it. Begin your day after throwing out the accumulated dirt from your body.

- Do not expose yourself to a draft after a warm bath. A sudden exposure to cold vitiates vata immediately.

Breakfast

It is recommended to have a warm and fluid breakfast with different kinds of porridge (dalia), halwas, and so on. Carrot halwa is highly recommended. For details of the recipes, you can consult my book: *Ayurvedic Food Culture and Recipes.*

Do not mix cold and hot things together. For example, some people in Europe eat yoghurt for breakfast and drink tea or coffee at the same time. You may drink tea or coffee half an hour before breakfast if you wish to eat yoghurt or fruits for breakfast.

Note: Those with various pains in the body should avoid eating yoghurt.

After breakfast, leaving the house...

Most people in the world start their workday after breakfast. Many have to leave the house and go somewhere else to study, to work, etc. Before leaving the house, touch a holy thing or a crystal or a stone and make a wish that you return healthy to your home. These little ceremonies help to make you tranquil and relaxed.

If you are driving to work, before starting your vehicle, take a deep breath and send the prana energy to your whole body. Take another deep breath and make a wish to put a cover of protection around your vehicle.

Frequently Asked Questions (FAQs) on the Morning Programme

Is your new programme FEEP enough to energise the body and all vital organs?

The idea to develop FEEP is based on the thinking that something is better than nothing. In my book, *Stress-free Work with Yoga and Ayurveda*, I have given a sixteen minute programme for a day. The reason to give FEEP is that people take it as seriously as brushing their teeth in the morning or going to the toilet. Certainly it is not enough; nevertheless it gives you a good start for the day. I suggest that if you can, do SN at least 5 times every morning. However, if you have constraints of time, do FEEP every morning and do SN on the weekends.

It is rather difficult to spend so much time in the morning to observe urine, stool etc., drink hot water and take an Ayurvedic bath. Is there any shortcut?
Reading this Section you might get the impression that it takes quite long to do this programme. In reality it is not so. The process of

learning and getting used to it is long. Gradually, it will become a part of your routine. An Ayurvedic bath may take 2 minutes more than your normal shower. Activities like massaging your toes and thumbs, pressing your ears or blowing your nose require only a few seconds each. Initially, the process of collecting the required things and then trying and remembering each step takes longer. If you like, you may start practising this routine on the weekends and then gradually incorporate it in your daily routine.

Instead of hot water or cardamom water, can one drink some kind of herbal tea or black tea or coffee in the morning?

Drinking hot water in the morning is for internal purification. Early morning, having rested the whole night, your stomach is empty. By drinking hot water, we wake up the system gradually and clean it at the same time. Hot water cleans or in a way rinses the entire alimentary canal as well as the urinary system. We all like to wash our eyes and rinse our mouths upon getting up. The internal parts of the body require something similar. Think of it just as you would not like to wash your external body with tea or coffee, similarly the internal body should also be purified with water. Water is the best purifier. If we drink some tea, coffee or orange juice, we make our digestive system work. Cardamom is added in water to make it a balanced drink. The quality of water varies from one place to another. Cardamom adds a little flavour and brings equilibrium to water. Cooked water is lighter to digest. In some Chinese methods, they add a little fresh ginger in the early morning water. Ginger does the same as cardamom if added in a small quantity (about one to two cubic centimetres in one litre of water).

MADHYAHNCHARYA—THE PROGRAMME AT WORKPLACE

Most of us spend a large part of our day at our workplaces or working in one form or another. In fact, when we leave out the sleeping hours, it turns out that we spend more time at work than at home. According to Ayurveda, the first priority of life should be desire for life. That means one should take care of one's health and well-being. The second priority of life should be to work in order to earn wealth. A long life without means of subsistence can be miserable. This is an extremely important theme and this entire book is focused on this subject. Here I will present briefly what you should incorporate in your day at work.

At your workplace, pay attention to the following:

- Begin your day with sattvic thoughts and wish for yourself a successful and fulfilling working day. Take five deep breaths before beginning your workday.

- Concentration is a very important factor. Direct all your mental and physical energy towards your work. Any problems related to home or something else should be kept aside temporarily.

- If you have problems at work with people or with the nature of work, make best of your efforts to take a tolerant approach to it. Try to think that nothing is perfect and that wherever there are groups of people, there are bound to be some problems. Try to endure in a sattvic manner. Do not suffer; either quit and change your work and if you cannot, then make an effort to alter your outlook and try to see the positive aspects of your situation.

- Many of you may have deadlines to meet. Fear of not meeting a deadline causes stress. Keep away from this fear as it diminishes work efficiency. Work with the idea in mind that what you are doing will be finished in the given time as it has to finish.

- To manage stress, take a break of about 30 seconds from time to time and do a special exercise which I have been inspired to devise for this purpose from Patanjali's Yogasutras. I like to refer to this exercise as PSAUV or "the five breaths exercise".

PSAUV for Stress Release

PSAUV is inspired from The Yogasutras of Patanjali. However, this specific exercise with five types of pranayama exercises in a row is not meant for the purpose of yoga. It is only inspired from Yoga for a quick relief from stress, tension and anger. 'P' is for prana, 'S' is for samana, 'A' is for apana, 'U' is for udana and 'V' is for vyana. You require about 30 seconds to do PSAUV.

1. **Prana** in technical language of Patanjali means breathing for the plexus region. That also denotes the physiological site of the breathing. Concentrate on your plexus region (the area around your heart) and send the breath there. Hold it a little and release gradually. After relieving the breath, wait for about 2 seconds for the next breath.

2. **Samana** literally means equal and in the technical language of yoga, it denotes the middle of the body, a point that divides the body into two equal halves: upper and lower. Concentrate on your navel region and send the second breath there. Hold it a little and release gradually. After relieving the breath, wait for about two seconds before the next breath.

3. **Apana** means lower or lower part of the body. For the third breath, bring your thoughts between the navel region and your feet and send the vital air to this area. Hold the breath a little and release it gradually. After releasing the breath, give a little pause before the fourth breath.

4. **Udana** means upper or rising. The fourth breath is guided to the head region. Let the vital air circulate in your head a little and then release it gradually. Give a little pause after releasing the breath.

5. **Vyana** means one of the three vital forces of the body and it is also called vata. This vital force, like the element air and ether it comes from, is everywhere in the body. For the fifth breath, visualise your whole body and let the vital air circulate in all parts of your body. Breathe gradually and send the air to head, shoulders and arms. Let the air circulate in your chest and abdomen and then to the legs. Breathe out gradually and stay still for about 3-4 seconds.

Keeping physical equilibrium

It is also important to have a correct posture while you are working. Pay attention to the following:

1. Always distribute your body weight equally on both sides when you are working, sitting or standing.
2. If you have a desk job, take care that you do not bend your shoulders and always sit straight.
3. For working, the tables should be at a convenient height. Always try and make some adjustments so that you do not strain your backbone by inconveniently high or low working surfaces.
4. During work breaks, do some stretching exercises given below.

Stretching exercises

1. Stretch back both your shoulders with strength. Your elbows are also pulled backwards in this process (Figure 46). Repeat this 2-3 times. You can do this exercise while sitting or standing.
2. Put both your hands behind your neck, clasp them and pull them back (Figure 47). Swing left and right in this position (Figure 48). This exercise can also be done sitting or standing.

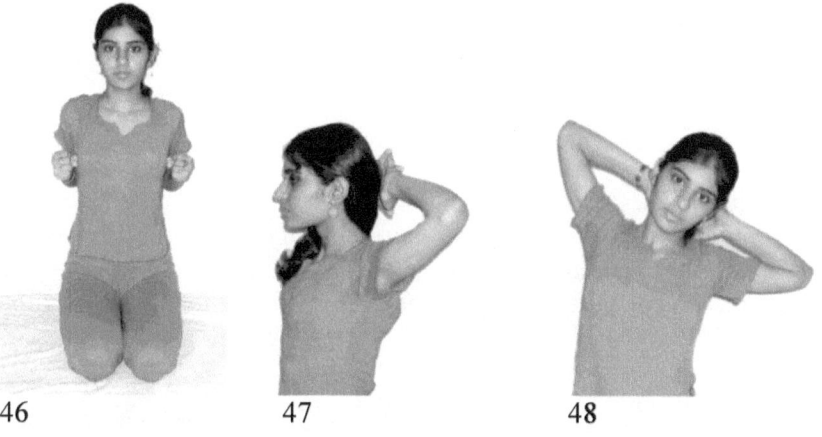

46   47   48

Stand up and stretch your body backwards and also put your hands backwards. Clasp your hands and stretch back (Figure 49). Swing left and right in this position.

3. Bend forwards, clasp your hands and stretch downwards while keeping your knees straight (Figure 50). Swing your body left and right.

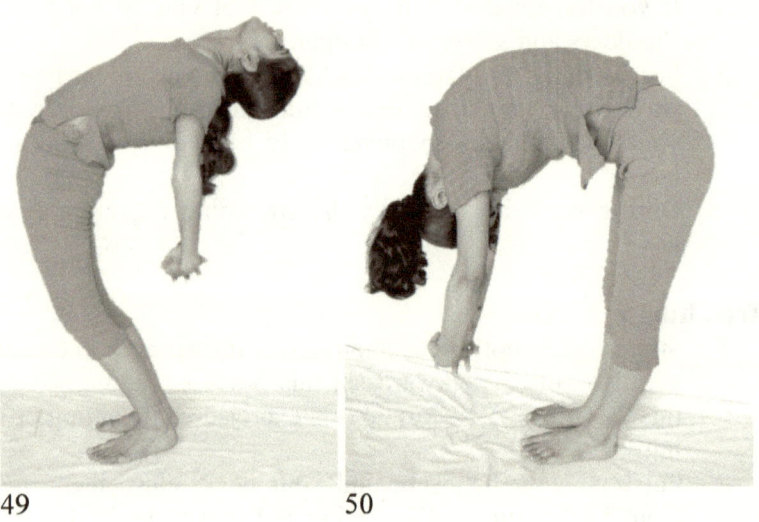

49   50

Note: You should do these stretching exercises as often as you feel you need to and the nature of your work allows. The first two exercises are also very useful if you are sitting in a plane or a train for a very long time as you can do them while sitting.

Lunch

According to the Ayurvedic principles, warm meals should be taken. The food products should be of good quality and fresh. Preserved foods and pre-prepared foods that are kept for a long time after preparation vitiate vata. Oils and other cooking mediums should be of good quality.

Many people in the world have their lunch at their workplaces. They either eat a cold lunch like sandwiches or eat in canteens. Canteens do provide warm food but the food products they use are usually not of good quality. Cold food taken in stress situations can be the cause of many health problems and can get ailments related to vata and pitta. To avoid all these, I suggest the following:

- If you are a sandwich eater, add some mixed salad in your sandwich along with the usual butter and cheese. Add some herbs like thyme, ajwain, dill seeds, etc. Buy always good quality bread that is freshly made. If possible, warm up your sandwiches. Try and drink something warm like herbal tea in small quantity during lunch. Choose the tea which has digestion promoting herbs like mint, mixed fruits, thyme, ajwain, ginger, basil, cardamom are some examples. If you do not like herbal teas, drink at least a cup of hot cardamom water.

- It is important to sit down before eating in order to rest a little and collect your thoughts in order to forget about the tension related to work. Either say a little prayer or wish yourself health and equilibrium with the food you are consuming or do PSAUV as described above. These few seconds of relaxing will make your food bring you the goodness of nature.

- After taking your food, make sure to rinse your mouth and eat two cardamoms. Cardamoms not only promote digestion but are also good for throat, voice, teeth and heart.

After concluding your workday, do the PSAUV once again and try not to take the worries of work home with you. Make a wish that you return back healthy to your workplace.

SANDHYACHARYA—THE EVENING PROGRAMME

Balancing the Workday

You should make an effort to balance your workday by doing activities in your spare time that are different from or even opposite to the nature of your work. For example if your work involves a lot of talking, telephoning and other such activities, you should have some quiet moments after your return from work. Wash your face, take a warm drink and lie down for about 15 minutes to half an hour in quietness. Do not listen to music, radio or television during this time. Your senses need complete rest from the vata activities they were involved in during the day. Those who travel or walk a lot or are working at a place that is loud, need a similar kind of rest.

Those of you who work alone and in closed rooms with computers, etc. need a refreshing walk in the evening to balance the heavy kapha energy that accumulates because of immobility.

Evening meal

The evening meal should be warm and of fluid in nature. It should not be heavy. It should not contain heavy foods like meat, lentils or foods cooked with large amount of fat. Fresh vegetable soups are highly recommended. Vegetable preparations cooked with a little fat are also good. Remember always to mix several vegetables together in order to make a holistic meal. The use of fresh ginger is highly recommended because it creates a balance of the three doshas and promotes digestion. Avoid hot chillies and eat spices like curcuma (turmeric), cardamom, cumin, coriander, clove, cinnamon, kalonji and fenugreek. Such spices are health-promoting and strengthen the immune system.

Some people eat a lot during the evening and go on eating other things even after having finished their dinner. These habits tend to give rise to numerous stomach ailments. If you eat something when your previous meal is in the process of digestion, you are doing harm to your stomach and ultimately to the whole system. According to Ayurveda, if we do that regularly, part of the partially digested food accumulates in our stomach. This ailment which is called *amadosha,* weakens the stomach and dirties the blood. Over a period of time, it gives rise to many skin ailments, allergies and digestive problems thus disturbing the whole system.

The evening meal should be taken at least two hours before going to bed. During these two hours, one should not eat anything, not even a chocolate or 'a little something'. It is not good for health to go to bed when digestion is still in progress. Thus, one should arrange dinner time according to one's sleep rhythm.

After-Dinner Walk

It is recommended that after dinner, one should go for a little walk. One should not sit or lie down after the evening meal. During the day, it does not matter so much but at night, body's *srotas* or energy channels slow down and therefore it is important to go for a walk in order to keep them open for the process of digestion. Besides that, to inhale fresh air in the evening, before going to bed is health promoting.

Entertainment

Many people, especially singles or couples without children go out a lot in the evening for entertainment, parties or cultural programmes. This is a very good way of diverting oneself from the routine work and to refresh oneself mentally. However, I have often observed that some people go out almost every evening and stay out until late. With the result, they start suffering from chronic fatigue. This is very bad for health. Each individual has a different level of stamina and it is important that you know your limits and find a balance between your health and entertainment.

Sleep

It is essential to get an appropriate quality and duration of sleep. For a normal adult, the sleeping time should be between 6 to 8 hours. Spiritually awakened persons can do with very little sleep of only a few hours. One should not sleep for more than 8 hours every day. Excessive sleep vitiates kapha and too little sleep vitiates vata. It is essential to create a pre-sleep atmosphere especially if you have trouble falling asleep. Prepare a silent atmosphere with dim lights before going to bed. Switch off radio or television and if you like to sleep with music, put on only meditative or soothing music. Speak very little and not too loud during this time.

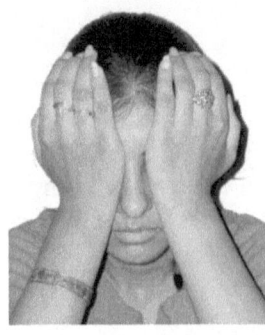

Care of the Eyes

Use some Ayurvedic or homeopathic eye drops to clean your eyes from the day's pollution. Relieve your eyes from the day's stress by pressing them gently with your palms. Put your palms on both your eyes and press gently in all directions (Figure 51). Move the palms up and down several times and then move them sideways.

Purification of the Mind

Purify your mind before sleep. During the day, through various activities, our minds are filled with people and actions. This is the rajas state of mind. There are also times when we are troubled with emotions like anger, jealousy or worry. This is the tamas state of mind. Make an effort to free your mind from all these thoughts and bring it to stillness. Make an effort to bring yourself to a sattva state of mind. Do some pranayama or simply PSAUV, the five-breath pranayama. Then concentrate on the darkness of night and on the stars and the moon. Repeat something like the following text in your mind:

O night's energy, you are there to rejuvenate us human beings. I pray to you to give my body a profound sleep. Bless me so that my senses and mind are at rest and I get a deep and rejuvenating sleep. Let my sleep be so restful that I wake up refreshed and healthy tomorrow morning. Give me an energising sleep. O nights energy, bless me with a sattvic sleep. Let me sleep like a yogi. Help me forget about the worldly things and let me sleep with a completely still and peaceful mind. O night's energy, bless me! I am grateful that you are there.

This example of a good night "prayer" is influenced by the mantras of Atharva Veda. You can make up your own text, repeat some mantra or do japa (repetition of a mantra) in any other form. In fact, repetition is very important here as it helps to empty the mind from rajasic and tamasic thoughts and brings stillness of mind.

RITUCHARYA RELATED TO DINCHARYA

Ritucharya means living according to the seasonal rhythm. According to Ayurveda, we have to take into account the changing seasons in our daily routine. Food is one of the very important factors in this direction. We have to balance our nutrition according to summer, winter, wet, dry and windy weather. Nutrition that is not according to the season leads to vikriti instantaneously. For example, some people go with this notion that they should eat certain particular substances because they are good for health. You should not do that without any regard to the season besides your prakriti. In the West, many people think that they should drink between 1 to 2 litres of water each day. The quantity of your water intake depends upon your food and season. If your food is prepared according to Ayurvedic principles and is fluid, you obviously need to drink less water. Similarly, the intake of water changes from hot to cold and dry to humid seasons. Thus, during cold and humid season, drinking excessive water will lead to kapha vikriti, will over-strain your kidneys and may lead to pain in the lower back.

Ayurveda recommends afternoon sleep only during summer months. Otherwise, sleeping during the day is not recommended. It can lead to kapha vikriti.

In brief, your daily routine should be moulded according to the Ayurvedic wisdom of nutrients and weather. These factors are discussed in the first chapter. For more information, you may consult my other books on related specific themes.

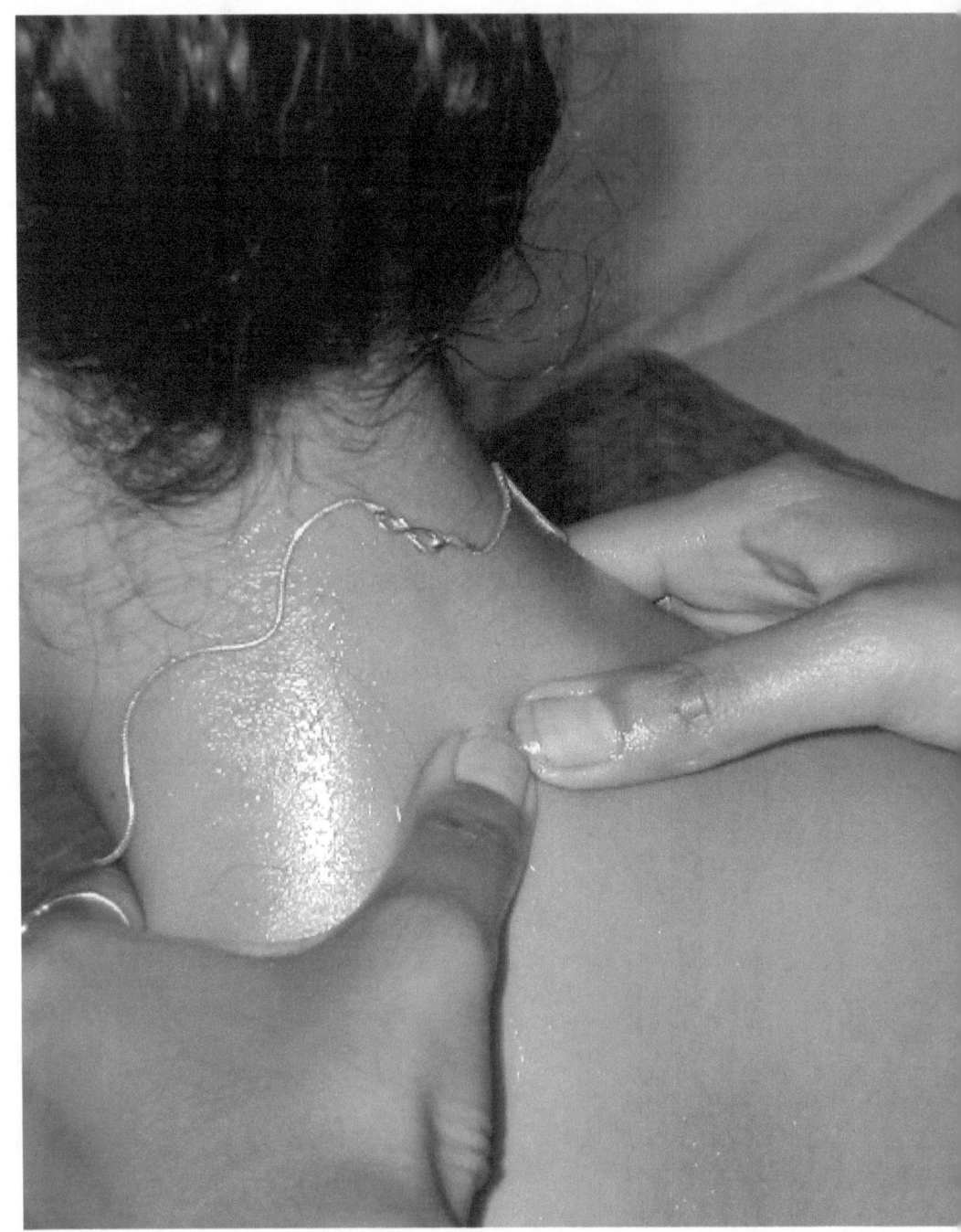

Chapter 4

Saptahcharya—The Weekly Programme

The weekly programme includes the following:

- Fasting
- Oil saturation body massage
- Head massage
- Vigorous face massage
- Hot bath or shower with etheric oils
- Chewing sesames seeds or mouth wash with sesames oil

WEEKLY PARTIAL FASTING DAY

According to Ayurveda, a complete fast vitiates vata and staying hungry is not advised. A semi-fast in the present context includes eating less and only selected food items. It is suggested that once a week, every week on the same day, you follow this altered regimen. Select a day and always keep the fast on the same day. You may choose any day of the week.

What to Eat on the Semi-Fast Day?

You can eat fruits, vegetables, nuts, yoghurt, milk and cheese. No preparations made of grains (e.g. rice, barley, wheat, maize, lentils, beans, etc.) and no salt should be taken on this day. The food should be sattvic and that means onions, garlic and other strong spices like chillies etc. should be avoided. Meat and eggs and anything else that is not vegetarian should not be eaten.

For breakfast you can have any of these things: cheese, nuts, fruits, carrot halva, yoghurt and milk. Your choice of cheese is restricted to the unsalted fresh cheese as most processed cheeses have salt in them.

If you have to work physically hard or walk a lot, you can have fruits like bananas and papaya or eat some nuts or cheese for lunch as well.

For the evening meal, you may prepare a plate of fresh vegetables by using some herbs and spices like cumin, ajwain or thyme, fennel seeds, ginger and cardamom. You can eat these with some potatoes but always remember not to add salt in it.

Benefits: This special diet once a week helps to purify the system and enhances self-control. If we eat in excess during the week or happen to eat something that does not suit the body, partial fasting helps to revitalise the digestive system. By eating less and eating things that have high water content, the system recovers from any trauma caused to it during the week. It is a kind of rest day for the digestive system.

The partial fast enhances self-control because there is one specific day a week when you eat your restricted diet. May be others around you are eating your favourite dishes or you may be passing by a market place with the smell of nice food and you have to learn to restrict yourself. This provides training to keep control on your senses. Control over your senses trains you to divert mind in the direction you wish.

Steps Two to Six of the Weekly Programme

The following six prescriptions are to be taken once a week or at least every 10 days according to your convenience. You need a session of about three hours a week to do all the six steps described below. These will renew your energy and give you a radiating and beautiful look. Despite being good looking, many people have a dull appearance and their complexion is not radiating and bright. It normally happens due to their hectic lifestyle, overwork and worries. This leads to vata vikriti and therefore one gets dull complexion and unattractive look. You will perceive an immediate effect of this treatment upon your looks and feelings. When vata is perturbed, the mind also wanders and one is unable to concentrate. Massage and warm treatment like fomentation or application of dry heat bring vata in equilibrium.

Oil Saturation Self Massage

As the name suggests, you have to apply oil to the body again and again until it is saturated with oil.

Choice of oil: Use different oils alternatively. Ghee, sesame oil, olive oil and coconut oil are some of the options. Ayurvedic massage oil can also be prepared by cooking powdered herbs in sesame oil. In some countries, oil from apricot seeds is available. It is a good oil for the skin. In any case, alternate the oil with ghee or coconut fat to nourish the skin and whatever you may use should be applied warm. Warm oil can penetrate the skin better and deeper.

There are numerous recipes for making Ayurvedic massage oils. Here is a very simple recipe so that you can prepare on your own with ease.

Preparation of Ayurvedic Massage Oil

Ingredients:

Fennel	50 gm (8 ounces)
Mustard seeds	50 gm (8 ounces)
Cress seeds	50 gm (8 ounces)
Liquorice	50 gm (8 ounces)
Sesame oil	1 litre (5 cups)

Crush all the ingredients into a fine powder and put them in one litre of hot sesame oil. Take care to use a pot of 5 litres for this purpose because when you add powdered herbs; the oil tends to boil over. For this reason, do not add the herbs in the fuming oil but it should be quite hot. However, it is important to heat the oil until it begins to fume. Then take it away from the heat and wait for about 30 seconds before adding the herbs. After adding the herbs, put the pot on re-duced fire and let it cook for about 5 minutes. Leave it like that overnight and the next day, filter the preparation through a cotton napkin. Squeeze out all the oil.

Body massage: Use a massage mat or an old blanket for doing massage. Heat up the oil or ghee in a bowl. You may keep the bowl in a hot water container so that it stays hot for a while. The oil should be applied to the body systematically and with forceful strokes so that the skin is able to absorb it. You can do the massage on your own or exchange with family or friends. I explain below various steps so that you can do the whole massage on your own including the back massage.

- With your right hand, massage the left hand and arm and do intensive massage especially on the joints.
- Massage each part a number of times and keep applying oil. Apply the oil by dipping your fingers in the oil container and then smearing it on various parts of the body (Figures 52-53).
- Massage the right hand and arm with the left hand in a similar manner.
- Massage the neck and ears and then descend to the shoulders (Figure 54).
- Massage the front part of the body now with both the hands by applying sufficient pressure and by repetitive strokes. Massage your face well and vigorously. Apply oil on your temples and massage them well (Figures 55-57).
- Massage your left leg from the feet to the pelvic joint and pay special attention to all the joints (Figure 58-59)
- Massage the right leg in a similar manner.
- Stand up and massage both hips well (Figure 60).
- Apply oil on your back (Figures 61-62). Some of you who do not have flexible bodies may have difficulty in doing so. In any case, if you are on your own, for massaging your back well, put a piece of plastic on your massage mat and smear oil on it. Lie down with your back on this plastic, bend your knees, put your thighs against your abdomen and hold your bent legs with your arms. Clasp both the hands together, lift your neck and rock your body backwards and forwards. Do that several times and then in the same posture rock sideways. (see figure 10 and 11 of FEEP) for making these movements.

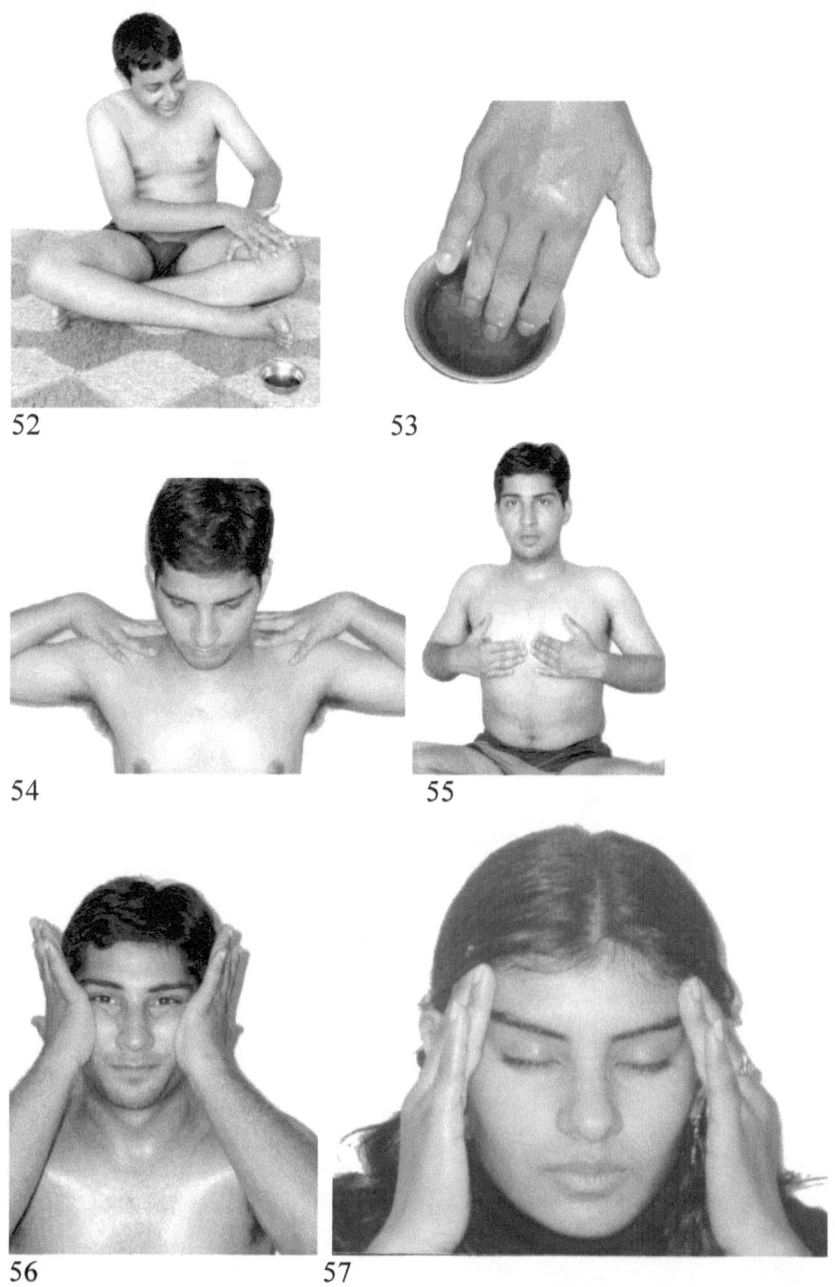

52

53

54

55

56

57

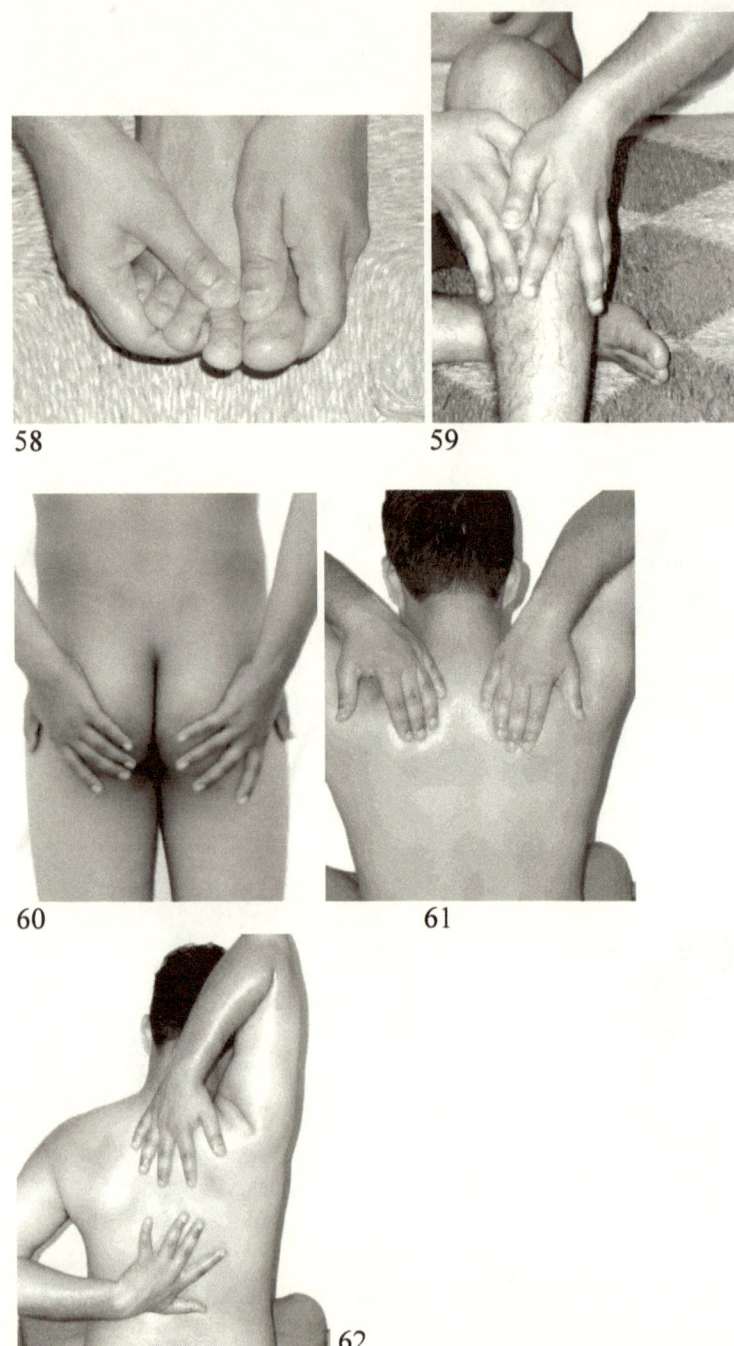

58

59

60

61

62

With the above eight steps, your body is oiled and massaged. Repeat the whole process two more times. You will require lesser oil for second and third time and your body will gradually get saturated with oil.

Head massage: Oil for massaging head is normally made with plants which are nerve soothing, promote hair growth and make it beautiful. Plants like Brahmi, Bhringraj, Ratanjot, Amala and Shikakai are used for this purpose. You may prepare this oil in a similar manner as the body massage oil but take only 5 gm of Ratanjot and 50 gm each of the rest of the plants. You may also use for head massage the same massage oil or pure coconut or olive or sesames oils.

On the head, the oil is applied at room temperature. Put some oil in a bowl and apply into the roots of the hairs with your fingers (Figure 63). Massage the scalp by moving your fingers. Once the scalp is oiled, massage it with both your hands simultaneously by moving your hands as you would do for playing a drum (Figure 64).

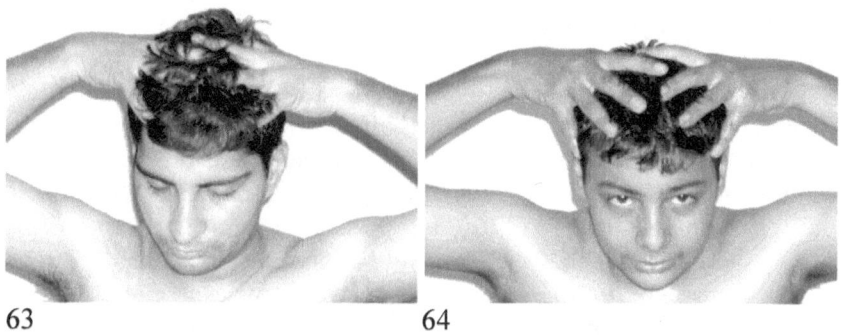

63   64

After the Massage

After your body and head massage, you can either leave the oil on yourself overnight or take a hot bath immediately afterwards. It is recommended to leave the oil at least for a few hours. In case you wish to leave it overnight, take a hand towel, wet it in hot water, squeeze it and wipe your body with it to take off the extra oil. After wiping off your body, you are able to dress up without spoiling your clothes with oil. But you will have to protect your pillow with an old towel from the oil in your hair.

Ayurvedic Herbal Bath

The purpose of bath is to apply wet heat on your body after the oil treatment. Extracts like rose water, a few drops each of Anise oil, Eucalyptus oil and Citronella may be added to this bath. If you are not familiar with these oils, you can add some commercial brands like amritanjan balm or Tiger balm or something similar in this category. Sit in the hot bath for 15 minutes to half an hour according to your need and convenience. After coming out of the bath, wrap yourself in a bathrobe and lie down for a short while. Make sure that there is no draft and you are well covered if it is cold weather.

Chewing sesames seeds or mouth wash with sesames oil

This last part of the weekly programme is not related to massage and bath and can be done at any time of the day. Sesame seeds should be chewed to strengthen the teeth and the inner cellular lining of the buccal cavity. Take black sesame seeds if possible. Put a teaspoonful of sesame seeds in your mouth. Chew them well for about 5 minutes and spit them out.

Alternatively, do *gandusha* or gargle with warm sesames oil. This protects the mouth and strengthens the inner lining. Take 1-2 teaspoons of warm sesames oil in your mouth and keep it there for about 5 minutes. Move it here and there with the air pressure so that it enters all the cavities between the teeth. Spit it out afterwards. In case you have trouble with teeth or gums or have blisters in mouth, you can do this as treatment. But for that, you are required to rinse your mouth with water after every meal and then do *gandusha* with sesames oil.

Chapter 5

Mahcharya—The Monthly Programme

The monthly programme includes the following:

- Purification of the mind
- Healing the body
- Special programme for women related to menstruation

The monthly programme does not need much of your time but it does need your attention. Principally it is for the mind. It is suggested that you make an inspection about your state of health every month. It is always better to deal with weakness and fatigue immediately rather than accumulate them. Women's life until a certain age centres around the monthly cycle, therefore, a special programme for them is given.

Purification of the Mind

Choose a day of the month and devote it to achieving mental purification by introspection. It is important to have a fix day every month for this activity. For example, choose 15th of each month or first or last Monday (or any other day) of the month. It is also a good idea to co-ordinate this day with your weekly fast day. Let us say that you fast on every Thursday. Then you can choose the first Thursday of every month for purifying your mind.

Purification of the mind is done by japa. Japa is the repetition of a mantra. The idea is to expel all the thoughts from the mind and attain a thought-free state of mind. It does not however mean that you cannot work on this day. Do your work as usual and let the mantra be at the back of your mind. It would mean that you begin chanting your mantra and go on doing it the whole day in your mind. Imagine you are at work, concentrating on preparing an urgent report. The mantra goes on at the back of your mind but the chain of the mantra is broken when a colleague of yours comes to discuss something and interrupts you. Afterwards you are perhaps still thinking about this conversation. Then react immediately and start repeating the mantra again.

Some of you may like to do a mantra or chanting silently the name of God. It is the same thing. Those of you who have a problem with God or mantra or both, may choose the sun. You may repeat the name of the sun in your own language or use one of the Sanskrit mantras for the sun, for example— Om Suryaye namah.

When you begin to repeat a mantra (or whatever else you choose) in the morning, after a while, it will start resounding automatically at the back of your mind. The idea of this practice is to break the chain of thoughts and silence the mind. You will also realise during this process that the mind wanders in so many diverse directions needlessly. By doing japa, we create a quieter inner environment.

In the evening of this particular day, take about twenty minutes for yourself and do some introspection of the events of the past month. Ask yourself questions like—were you good to yourself? Were you compassionate to others? Were you satisfied with yourself? Did you have inner peace? Did you entertain tamasic thoughts like jealousy, anger, excessive attachment or greed? Try and work on yourself from the type of answers you get from the above questions.

Try and live with the idea of 'forget and forgive'. Have compassion and love for other human beings around you. Nevertheless do not be weak or cowardly. Cultivate courage in yourself. Develop your communication skills. Do not keep things in your mind and feel guilty or angry at others. The idea of this monthly programme is to learn not to suppress emotions or bad feelings. Suppression leads to formation of deposits of tamas inside the mind and sooner or later gives rise to disorder in the body or mind. Doing japa or using some other method to silence your mind brings you in a profounder state of consciousness, and solutions to the problems you are facing come to the surface automatically.

Healing the Body

If you are a healthy person, the daily and the weekly programmes are enough to maintain your health. Nevertheless, it is essential to do self-examination during the monthly programme. It is possible that you have had special situations like too much travelling or some other stressful event that affected you. Normally in such circumstances, vata is vitiated. You may have symptoms like fatigue, constipation, restless sleep, dry throat and dry skin. If these symptoms do not go away after the weekly programme (massage and warm bath), you may need to apply an enema with fat. Enemas are explained in the half yearly programme. Only in special circumstances do you need to apply the fat enema in your monthly programme.

It is always good to take care of the disorders and imbalances instantaneously. If you leave them unattended, they take a serious turn. For example, if you do not attend to the initial symptoms of vata vitiation, you will get stiffness in the body and various kinds of aches and pains. The longer an imbalance remains, the harder it becomes to re-establish the equilibrium. To cure vitiated vata, do the oil saturation massage, warm bath, appropriate rest and take sweet and unctuous food.

Symptoms of vitiated pitta may appear in the form of skin rupturing, blister, herpes and indigestion. You may feel excessive heat in your body. Stop taking sour, salty and pungent foods and treat yourself with one of the bitter teas.

A sweet taste in your mouth, too much sleep and sticky stool are the symptoms of kapha vitiation. To cure it, do some exercise, take warm treatments like a vapour bath and eat spicy and sour foods.

Normally, the imbalance of the vital energies should be attended to immediately. But I am mentioning this in the monthly programme as well because in case you have been ignoring yourself, the monthly programme is the opportunity to attend to any vikriti of one or more doshas. The older you are, the more alert you have to be with respect to vikriti and more effort is needed to recover to prakriti. When we are still young, somewhere between 17 and 45 years of age, the body can tolerate a lot because it has the maximum ojas (immunity and vitality).

Due to the high ojas, the recovery from vikriti to prakriti is easier and faster than when we are older. If we let the vikriti dwell, it gradually gives rise to various minor disorders. These disorders, if not attended to, become either chronic or cause a serious ailment. Thus, monthly attention to the activities of our body and mind is extremely essential to keep a check on our state of health.

Menstruation

A woman's life revolves around menstruation during the reproductive period. During menstruation, disorders are thrown out of the body and a woman regains balance. The extent of suffering during menstruation denotes the imbalance or stress she has had during the month. I have described all this in detail in my book, *The Kamasutra for Women*. In the present context, I want to convey that women should observe their menstruation well and should diagnose themselves. A stressful month with a hectic lifestyle gives rise to troublesome menstruation. If you have a peaceful and quiet time, the menstruation is also smooth. If you always have trouble during menstruation, then you need specific treatment. I am describing below some diagnostic methods so that you can clearly ascertain your body's state.

1. Dark brown blood or reduced quantity of blood or both these factors together indicate vata vitiation.

2. Excessive blood indicates pitta vitiation (if it is not due to some gynaecological disorder)

3. Pink blood with a lot of mucous is indicative of kapha vitiation

A little before and during menstruation, notice your symptoms carefully and interpret them as follows:

1. Constipation before menstruation indicates vata imbalance. If the constipation persists until the menstruation begins, it becomes the cause for pain.

2. If you get mild diarrhoea, it means you have had pitta imbalance and the body throws out this imbalance in this manner.

Sickness and vomiting indicate kapha imbalance. By vomiting, the system purifies itself and gets rid of the kapha imbalance.

Measures: In case of constipation, take warm and liquid foods, have physical exercise, and drink hot water in the morning to ensure proper evacuation

In case of diarrhoea or vomiting do not take any medication to prevent them. They are just a part of the cleansing process. Nevertheless, if you have these symptoms, make sure that you take measures to maintain your equilibrium. You can do that with nutrition, yoga and other minor alterations in your lifestyle as is suggested in the daily and weekly programmes.

Note: If you have more complicated troubles than just due to the imbalance of doshas, it is essential to get proper treatment. I have described many remedies in my book, The Kamasutra for Women. It seems that in modern medicine, there is not much to help women with menstrual troubles. Generally hormones are prescribed. On the other hand, in Ayurveda and homeopathy, there are many valuable remedies to help women with menstrual troubles and menopause.

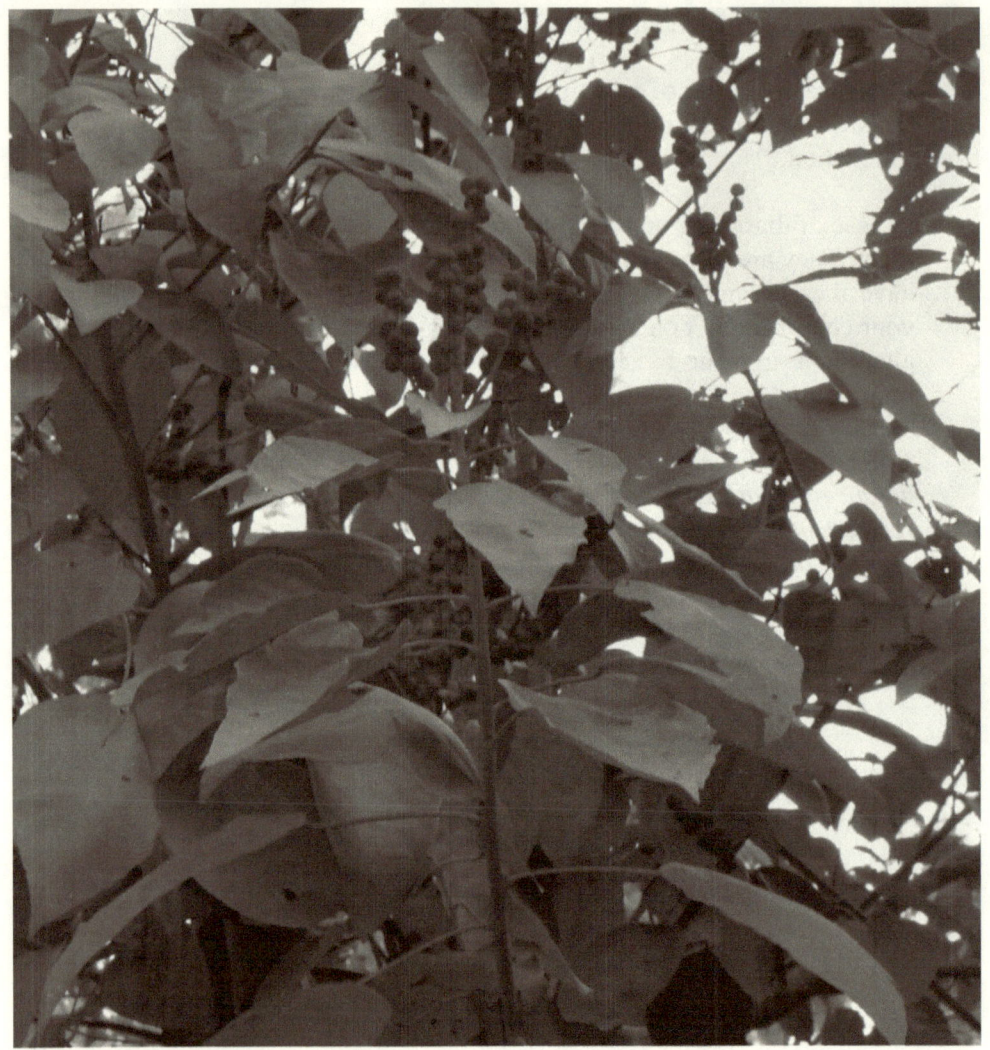

Kamala tree

Chapter 6

Sharirshuddhi—The Half Yearly Purification

Urban population all over the world spends a tremendous amount of money to make their appearances impressive and to maintain their houses, gardens, cars, etc. However, they do not think of rejuvenating their bodies and minds with similar enthusiasm and zeal. Several rich people regularly change their furniture, curtains and many other household things to give a new look to their homes. This concept of renovation in the sense of rejuvenation should also be applied to the human body and mind. If you are working very hard in your office or business, you always need a respite after about three months and require a change of environment. Sometimes, even after a short break of 3-4 days, one feels stronger and rejuvenated. In a similar manner, the body needs a break from the routine and needs to be purified about every six months. Half-yearly inner cleaning and care revitalise the body and gives it a good appearance, better resistance, high vitality and longevity.

It is easier to understand why there is a need to clean inner parts of the body if you can visualise them like the external parts. All of us pay enormous attention to the cleaning and hygiene of the external body parts. When you get up in the morning, you would not begin your day without washing your eyes or rinsing your mouth. Similarly, you would feel refreshed each morning after a shower or a bath. Inner parts of the body also need cleaning and care from time to time just like the external ones. You would immediately feel the effect of not cleaning the external body parts. Similarly, if we do not clean the internal parts of our body, diverse imbalances, aches, pains or disorders occur. With regular cleaning and care, the internal organisms continue to function efficiently.

Inner cleaning of the body is important to throw out the toxins we consume from sprayed foods grown with fertilisers and preservatives used to increase the shelf life of the food. The poisons may be in the form of biological infections, antagonistic food or artificial fertilisers, pesticides, consumption of chemical drugs, and so on. For a healthy and long life, it is absolutely essential that we purify ourselves periodically and get rid of these substances. The 'inner dirt' is subtler than the outer or the visible dirt because we do not know about it until it manifests itself in the form of disorders. We can compare these two to the dirt on the clothes and stains on them. The dirt goes away quickly with soap and water, but to remove the stains is more complicated.

INNER CLEANING PRACTICES OF AYURVEDA, YOGA AND THE TRADITIONAL CEREMONIES

The Ayurvedic inner cleaning practices are called **Panchakarma** (the five cleaning practices). Considering the range of undesirable chemicals we consume in our times, I have added two more practices and made it **Saptakarma** (the seven cleaning practices).

Besides the traditional cleaning practices of Ayurveda, there are also a number of cleaning practices of yoga and there are nutritional methods of self-cleaning which are part of the ceremonial Hindu tradition. These latter are the easiest to apply. I will describe here the three types of cleaning practices and you can choose according to your time and convenience. However, the most complete purification is done with Saptakarma.

Time for Inner Cleaning Practices

The inner cleaning practices should be done twice a year after the two principal seasons—winter and summer. During the cold and hot seasons, the body tends to accumulate an imbalance of doshas and thus, spring and autumn are the times to purify it and get rid of these imbalances. Mid-March to mid-April and mid-September to mid-October are the times to purify oneself. In fact, the Navratra fasts are also during this period and are meant for the purification of the body and mind. Thus, the medical need is imbibed in ceremonial tradition.

Navratra—The Nine-Days Fast

Navaratra literally means 9 holy nights. According to the Vedic moon calendar, they fall on the rising moon for the first nine days during the month of Chaitra (around mid March) and the month of Ashwin (around mid September). The ritualistic symbolism of Navratra is to worship the nine different forms of the goddess Shakti or Durga (the power). This is quite appropriate from the biological and medical point of view as all these rituals, ceremonies and fasts enhance mental and physical power and rejuvenate the body. The body is purified through special regimen and the mind is strengthened with sattvic thoughts and japa.

As I have already pointed out in the weekly programme, a complete fast is prohibited in the Ayurvedic scriptures as it vitiates vata. During navratra, a partial fast with a special regimen is recommended which is quite like the weekly fast except that here you can eat rock salt (sendhav salt). The rules for the nine-day fast are as follows:

- Foods made of grains like wheat, barley, maize, lentils, chickpeas etc. should not be eaten. Eat fruits and milk products instead. Have only two meals a day. Breakfast is light with fruits, nuts and milk or something similar. Soya milk is ruled out since Soya is a grain.

- Dry fruits like almonds, raisins, coconut and so on can also be taken.

- You may eat fruits or yoghurt etc. in between two meals in case you are doing physical activity.

- The second meal can be taken in the evening. You can eat potatoes, vegetables, cheese etc. In India, there are several replacements of grain flour that can be used to make a kind of bread. These flours are made from the tiny fruits of certain plants. They are commonly sold in food shops during the period of Navaratra.

- The food should not be prepared with onions, garlic or other spices that excite the senses. You may use spices like cumin, fennel, cardamom, clove, cinnamon and fresh ginger. Use a very

111

moderate quantity of salt and prepare the food with a little amount of fat.

• Do not eat too many sour fruits. Include bananas and papayas in your menu.

For the first two to three days, you may feel hungry or it may seem difficult to control yourself when others are enjoying big meals around you. However, on the third or fourth day, you will get used to it and your body will find a balance with the reduced quantity of food.

In addition to the special diet, it is suggested to cultivate sattvic thoughts like love, compassion, kindness and so on during this period and control tamasic thoughts related to ill feeling towards others, anger, jealousy and desire. Doing japa (silent repetition of a mantra) in the morning and evening is recommended. You may use any other mode of concentration or meditative practice.

The nine-days fasting makes you feel healthy and active. Those of you who sleep too much, have a weary feeling, or are slightly overweight (symptoms of kapha vitiation), will feel particularly good.

If you have excessive heat in your body or are suffering from other pitta vitiation symptoms, you may get a mild diarrhoea during this period that throws out the extra heat and creates a balance.

Those with symptoms of vata vitiation will have proper evacuation, flexible body and will feel calm due to the nine-day sattvic food and way of life.

After nine days of partial fast and sattvic thoughts, the body and mind attain their equilibrium again. This method of purification is not so intensive as the yogic and the Ayurvedic cleaning practices, but it offers you a choice which is lesser time consuming than the other two types of cleaning practices. If you cannot spare the time required for one of the complete programmes, at least stick to this simple way of purifying yourself every six months.

Yogic Cleaning Practices

Yogic purification practices are for adepts of yoga. We should keep in mind that the body of an adept of yoga is generally cleaner than others because they observe a special sattvic diet and eat very little. With the yogic purification practices, they purify the body further. Besides, due to yogasanas and pranayama, the adept's body and mind are constantly purified.

There are hundreds of purification practices described in different bodies of yogic literature. For this book, I have selected some of those which you can do on your own. I describe below five major practices and also give a schedule for each practice.

Jala Neti (Cleaning the nose with water)

Jala means water and it is a practice for cleaning the nasal passages with water. It should be done in the morning before breakfast. It is done with a neti pot which is a small pot with a nozzle. Fill this pot with clean drinking water. Take warm water with a pinch of rock salt

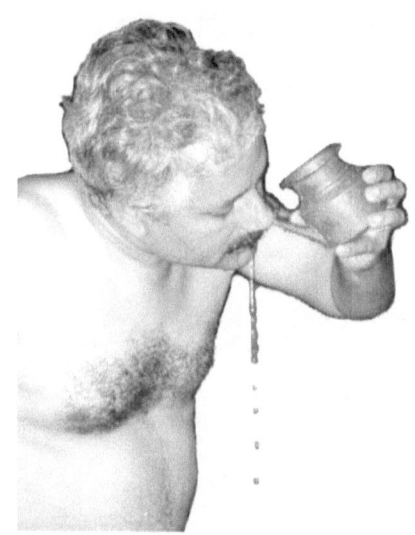

in it (0.1%). Hold the pot in your right hand. Tilt your head slightly backward, then to the left side and then slightly forward. Relax and start breathing through your mouth. Insert the nozzle of the pot into your right nostril and tilt it gently so that the water flows through the right nostril to the left (Figure 65). The water should flow smoothly until the pot is empty. Then blow your nose in order to clear the nasal passages. Repeat the same from the left to the right nostril.

65

After this practice, it is possible that you have water coming from your eyes, nose and mouth. Some phlegm may also come out from your nose and throat. All this depends upon the extent of blockage you have in the upper region. After a few days of regular practice, the passage will be clear and you will be able to breathe smoothly.

Do this exercise for a week in the beginning. Once the nasal passage is clear, you may reduce the frequency to once or twice a week. If you live in polluted areas or you tend to have frequent attacks of cold, it will be beneficial to do this practice daily.

Jala Dhauti (Washing the stomach with water)

Drink ¾ to 1 litre of hot water with a pinch of rock salt on an empty stomach in the morning. Move around for about a minute and then vomit out the water by bending down at an angle of 45^0 and tickling your throat with your fingers (Figure 66). The water will come out in 4 to 5 impulses. Do not do more than 8 impulses. This practice purifies the stomach, trachea and throat.

Your posture is extremely important when doing jala dhauti. Do not bend too much as it is harmful for the stomach. Washbasin is generally too low, so make some other arrangements for this practice. For example, you can take a stool and put a container on it. Bending too much while throwing out hurts the stomach. (Figures 67).

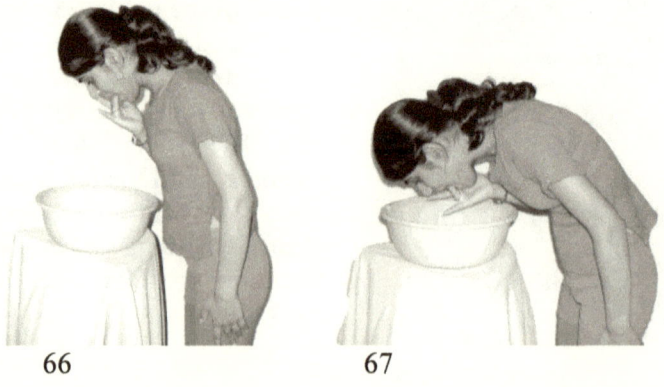

66   67

If your stomach is healthy, the water that is thrown out has the same taste as you drank it. If you have problems vomiting and you feel that your body has absorbed all the water very quickly, you have vata vitiation. In this case, repeat the practice the next day and drink a glass of normal water before drinking salted water for vomiting out. Bitter or sour taste in the vomited water indicates pitta vitiation. A light and balanced diet and repeated practice of jala dhauti will be beneficial in this case.

If you vomit too much or the water is foamy or slimy, it indicates kapha vitiation. You need to pay attention to your diet and repeat this practice for several days.

If you throw out food from the previous day, you are suffering from amadosha and a proper treatment is required.

If you are healthy, you may do jala dhauti once a week. It helps to keep a check on the condition of your health.

In case of imbalance, take other precautions to regain the balance and do this practice twice a week. In case of amadosha, do jala dhauti daily for about two weeks and eat a very simple and restricted diet like boiled vegetables and rice, a little freshly made yoghurt, fruits like papayas, sweet grapes and bananas. In case the problem persists, consult a physician.

Antara Dhauti (Purification of the alimentary tract)

This practice is for the purification of the alimentary tract. Take about 3 litres of drinking water. Heat the water and add half a teaspoon of rock salt. Bring yourself to a completely relaxed state and begin drinking water. After drinking the first half litre of water, do the following exercises.

- Stand straight, stretch both your arms upwards and clasp your hands. Make circular movements from your waist (Figure 68). All the upper parts of the body, including your stretched out arms are involved in this movement. With this exercise, you will feel the movement of the water in your stomach. Make five to seven rounds clockwise and an equal number anticlockwise.

Sit down, relax again and drink another half litre of hot salted water. Then do the following exercises.

- Stand up and put both your hands on your waist and make circular movements from the waist (Figure 69). You are moving the lower part of the waist as compared to the above exercise. You can feel the water moving in the intestines. Take about 5 rounds in each direction.

- Relax once again and drink a cup of water (¼ litre). Sit on your feet while your arms are stretched forward and your elbows rest on your knees (Figure 70).

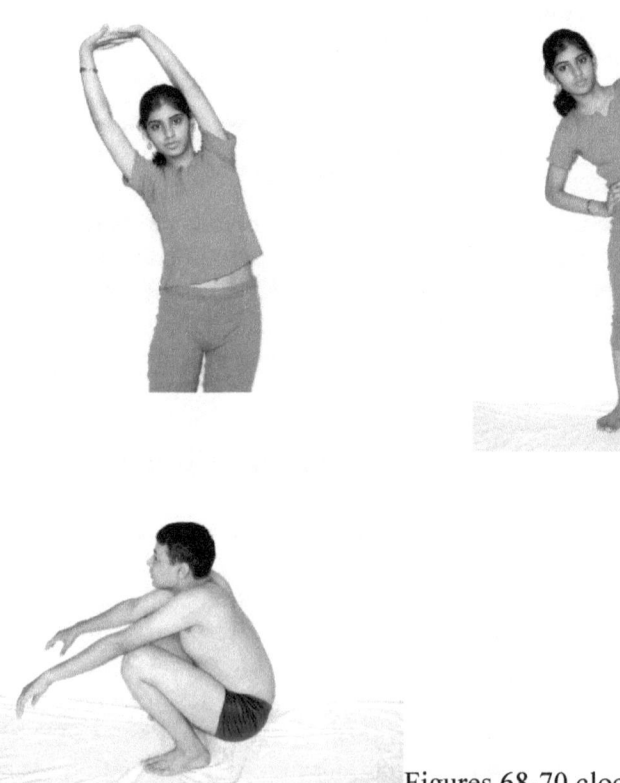

Figures 68-70 clockwise

Most of you will have an urge to go to the toilet by this time. You will pass both urine and faeces several times. Drink two more times half litre of water and each time sit on your feet as above. In the end, your intestines will be completely cleaned and only the water will pass through the anal passage.

After Antara dhauti, it is important to lie down and rest. Drink some herbal tea made with one teaspoon of fennel, about 10 basil (Tulsi) leaves and 4-5 crushed cardamoms in 1 litre (5 cups) of water. Bring to boil and cook it covered on a low heat for about 5 minutes. For lunch, have liquid foods like porridge, gruel or a soup. In the evening, eat some light preparation of rice like khichari. Do not do heavy work or anything hectic for the following two days.

This practice should be done every six months and not frequently.

Jala Basti (Water enema)

Basti means enema. Yogic basti is different from the Ayurvedic basti. In fact, the name basti comes from Ayurveda as the water is injected through the anal passage and the container that was used to hold water in former times was the bladder of animals. Bladder is called 'basti' in Sanskrit. But in yogic basti, the container is not used.

Sit down in a tub of warm water and try to get the water inside through the anal passage by moving its muscles. Shrink and relax the anal muscles again and again and the water will go in. Do this for about half an hour with pauses in between. Come out of the water, wrap yourself in a towel or gown and lie down on a mat while taking care that there is no air draft. Lift up your legs gradually one by one. After few minutes, get up and walk around gently. Sometimes during this process, you will have a strong urge to let the water out. You will have to go to the toilet several times. Faeces, water and some wind will be thrown out. After doing jala basti, take the same precautions with food and rest as after antara dhauti.

Jal Basti should also be applied every six months. Make sure that it is applied at least one week after antara dhauti.

Kapalabhati

Kapalabhati is a pranayama practice meant to purify the head region. It is a very simple practice you can do in about two to three minutes. It can also be used to achieve concentration and attain peace of mind.

Do this practice in the open air or at least with a window open to get fresh air. Sit down in a comfortable posture and start breathing very fast as you do when you are running. You are breathing very fast and at times through your nose and at other times through your mouth. It is like being 'breathless' after running up a flight of stairs or doing some other strenuous exercise. After a short while, you will feel tired and automatically stop breathing for a few moments. You will get a feeling of coolness in your head region and you will stay completely still. You can repeat this three times after a short interval.

If you like, you can do this practice every day. It helps to improve your memory and enhances the power of concentration by opening the energy channels in the head region. Do at least once a week to purify the head region.

Caution: If you are weak or anaemic, or have any cardiac problem, do not do this practice. Also avoid it shortly before menstruation, as some of you may feel giddy.

Ayurvedic Cleansing Practices: The Saptakarma

There are seven cleansing practices that should be done every half year. You need some special preparation before starting these practices called purvakarma. Similarly, you have to take special care after the completion of each practice and that is called pashchatkarma. Figure 71, gives an overview of these practices.

I give you the simple and modified version of these practices so that you can do them on your own every six months. For example, the classical nasya or head-cleaning practice cannot be done without the help of a physician. I have done research and have devised an alternative method that you can easily do on your own.

The classical purification practices of Ayurveda are not only used for the half yearly cleansing, but are also extensively used as therapeutic measures to cure various ailments. Different kinds of medicated enemas are applied to cure diverse ailments. The principal purpose is to detoxify the body from all the impurities and from the outside agents that hinder the natural functions of the system.

It is important that you plan these cleansing practices carefully in order to complete them without taking any extra time off from work. For the first four, you need three weekends and for the seventh practice (diuresis) also you need an afternoon free. The fifth and sixth practices can be integrated in your free time in the evenings or whenever you have time on working days.

For purvakarma, you need about 10 evenings. On the following four weekends, you can complete the other practices. I have given a time schedule for all the practices for your facility.

Schedule for Saptakarma

Purvakarma (the pre-treatment)

Purvakarma has three major elements: massage, fomentation and drinking fat. In fact, oil massage and drinking fat are under the category of snehan, which means application of fat. Massage or abhiyanga is of two kinds- with fat (snehan abhiyanga) or without fat (pressure massage. Those with kapha disturbances should be given pressure massage instead of oil massage.

The Purvakarma massage is the same as in the weekly programme. During ten days of purvakarma, do the oil saturation massage thrice. Fomentation is done after the massage as described below.

Fomentation or **sweating** is done in two forms—wet and dry. Massage should be done before fomentation.

Figure 71. A summary of Saptakarma

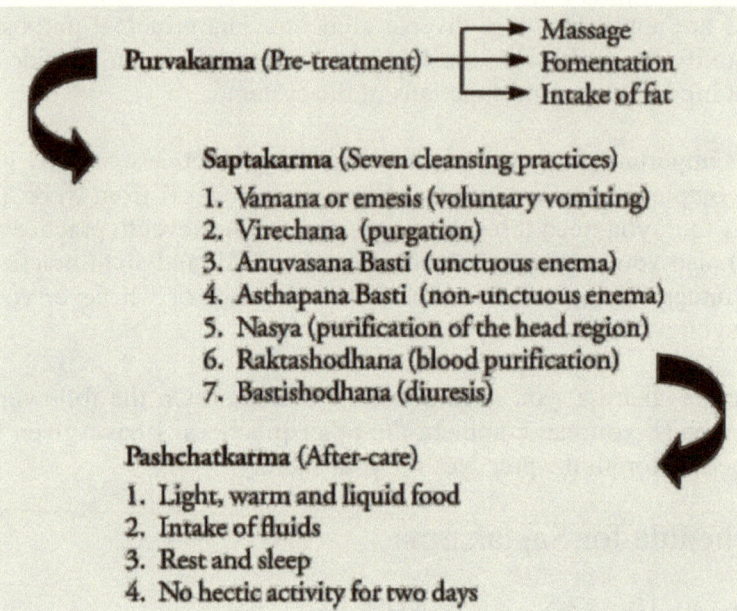

Purvakarma (Pre-treatment) → Massage
→ Fomentation
→ Intake of fat

Saptakarma (Seven cleansing practices)
1. Vamana or emesis (voluntary vomiting)
2. Virechana (purgation)
3. Anuvasana Basti (unctuous enema)
4. Asthapana Basti (non-unctuous enema)
5. Nasya (purification of the head region)
6. Raktashodhana (blood purification)
7. Bastishodhana (diuresis)

Pashchatkarma (After-care)
1. Light, warm and liquid food
2. Intake of fluids
3. Rest and sleep
4. No hectic activity for two days

Wet fomentation can be easily done in a bathtub. For dry fomentation, you need to overheat a small room with heaters. Alternatively, if you have a possibility of building a little fibreglass room on the roof or in the garden, you can make an excellent fomentation chamber heated by the sun. This chamber can be as small as 1m 20 (4 feet) on each side and should be built in the form of a pyramid for enhancing the absorption of sunrays (see box for details).

Dry fomentation is done by sitting inside the pyramid or a heated chamber in the afternoon as by then it has heated up with the sun. Keep something to drink with you. Stay for about 3-4 minutes after you start sweating. The time it takes before you begin to sweat depends upon your constitution. Wrap yourself well before coming out of the pyramid and stay indoors while you are sweating. Take care that there is no draft. Lie down and rest until you are completely dry.

Construction of a Pyramid for Dry Fomentation

The pyramid is easily made by joining four triangular wooden frames of appropriate dimensions. The tips of the triangles join at the top (see figure 53). I give below the proportion of each triangle and from that you can calculate other sizes.

Width: 72 cm (28.8 inches)
Sides: 68 cm (27.2 inches)

The narrow side of the each triangle is on the top. Remember that the above measurements are not the space between two pieces of wood, but also include the width of the wood for measuring the base of the triangle. Pieces of fibreglass are nailed on this frame with a baton on them. Cover all the frames completely with fibreglass. You need to make a door in one of the triangles.

You need a compass for an exact placement of the pyramid. The four faces of the pyramid face each direction. That means the corners of the pyramid are facing the four angles the four directions make with each other. The face with the door should be towards east. If for some reason, it is not possible, then keep it towards north.

According to our ancient scriptures, there are in total ten directions. The four main directions as we all know, four angles the four directions make with each other, and the upward and the downward directions. In Sanskrit, we have names for the four angles the four major directions make with each other. Northwest is called vayavya, northeast is called ishan, southwest is naitritya and southeast is called agnaiya. Ancient Hindu architecture or Vastu is designed in relation to the ten directions. The shape of the pyramid is such that it draws maximum energy from all the ten directions of the cosmos. Thus, the pyramid is not only meant for fomentation, but also for healing and energising the body.

Figure 72. A sketch of the directions of the cosmos and the pyramid

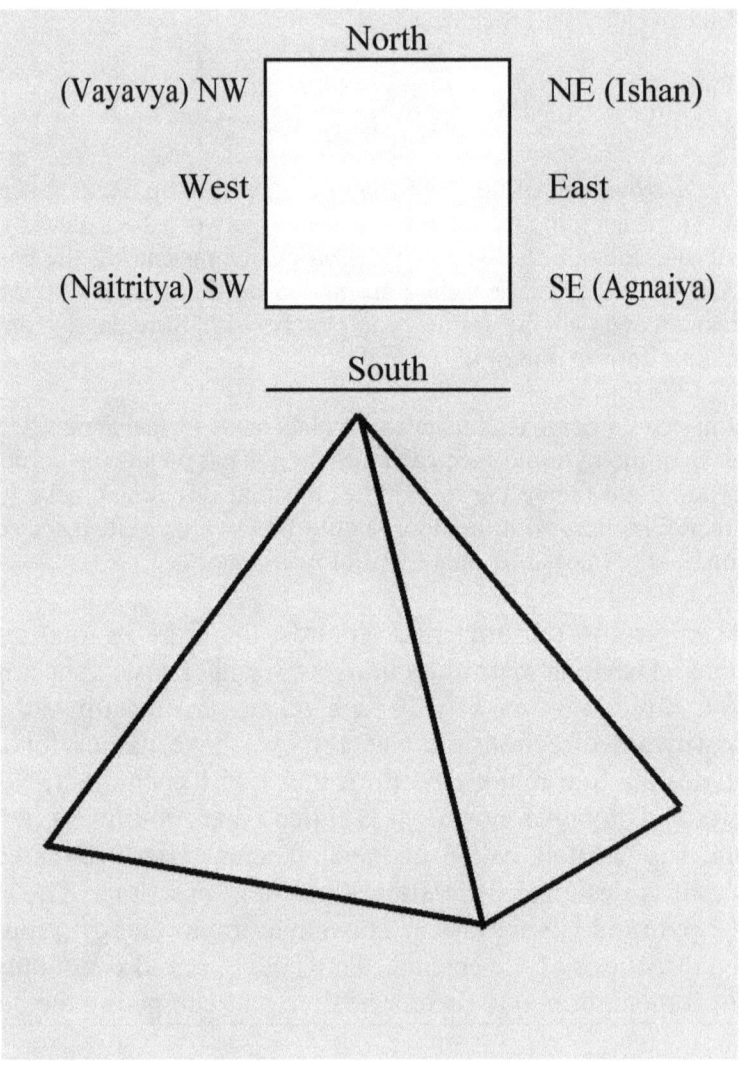

Wet fomentation: Prepare a hot bath with some etheric oils like anise oil, eucalyptus oil, citronella oil, rose essence or lemon grass oil. Add a few drops of each of these oils. If you are not familiar with these oils, you just add a tiny bit of Tiger balm or Amritanjan balm. Sit in the bath until you begin to sweat. If it takes too long before you start sweating and the water is getting cooler, add more hot water. After you begin sweating, come out of the bath, wrap yourself in a towel or a bathrobe and go to a pre-prepared warm bed with a hot water bottle. Keep a thermos with hot tea bedside. Take some tea and lie down for a while. With all these warm measures, you will continue to sweat. Keep lying sown until the sweat is completely dried. Make sure that you are not exposed to any draft in your bath or in your bedroom.

Caution: There is loss of fluid from the body during fomentation, therefore drink plenty afterwards. Take some rest after fomentation. Do not do fomentation in excess as it causes weakness and fatigue.

Fat drinking: After you are finished with your massage and fomentation, drink butter fat (ghee) for the following three days before going to bed in the doses given below. Either take the melted ghee as such or whip it in some hot milk along with some candy sugar. If you do not drink milk, have the ghee in a clear vegetable soup.

- Day 1: Three teaspoons
- Day 2: Five teaspoons
- Day 3: Eight teaspoons

Caution: Fat or obese persons or those with vitiation of kapha should not drink fat.

A Complete Schedule of Purvakarma

- Day 1: Massage and dry or wet fomentation
- Day 5: Massage and wet or dry fomentation
- Day 7:   Massage
- Days 8 to 10:   Fat drinking

Saptakarma

As described earlier, in saptakarma, you do seven purification practices spread over a period of about four weeks. They could be done in shorter time but I have made the schedule in such a way that working people can do the major practices over the weekends.

Caution: Saptakarma practices should not be done if you are unwell, feel weak, are pregnant or are convalescing after an ailment.

1. Vamana or Emesis

Vamana is a form of voluntary vomiting, similar to *Jala Dhauti* which I already mentioned in the Yogic purification practices. But it is a much more powerful and intensive purification procedure and therefore is done only once every six months, whereas *Jala Dhauti* can be done every week. The main feature of *Vamana* is a decoction of special herbal mixture which you drink in very large quantities.

Vamana is one of the major treatments to bring the equilibrium of kapha.

Decoction for vamana

Powdered liquorice (mullathi)	2 tablespoons
Water	1 ½ litre (7 ½ cups)
Rock salt	1 teaspoon

Add powdered liquorice in boiling water and cook with the lid on for about 15 minutes on a low fire. At the end, add salt into it and filter through a fine strainer or cheesecloth.

A very effective Ayurvedic drug for vamana is Madana phala called Emetic nut in English (*Randia spinosai* in Latin). The dose for vamana is 1 to 2 gm. There are many methods to take it but my preferred one is to mix one gram with the above decoction.

Drinking and vomiting: Vamana is done in the morning after getting up. First, drink your usual hot water with cardamom. After about ten minutes, drink the hot vamana decoction. Normally, after drinking about ¾ of a litre (4 cups), you already feel like vomiting. In case you do not, drink a little more, wait for about ten minutes and then induce vomiting by tickling in the throat with your finger. Take care that the angle for vomiting is 45^0 and not 90^0. That means that you should not bend too low (see Figures 66-67).

Normally, when vomiting is initiated, the other impulses follow after the first vomit. Try to have up to six impulses but never more than eight.

Results: This process thoroughly cleans out the upper part of the digestive tract, principally the stomach. Depending upon your condition, you may throw out the decoction in different forms and get rid of diverse imbalances.

If you are healthy and have no imbalance, the liquid will come out in the same state as you took it in. It is like pouring something into a clean glass and then emptying it again.

If it is difficult for you to vomit and you belch a lot, it means that you have vata vitiation. Throwing up liquid with a bitter or sour taste is a sign of pitta vitiation. This kind of vomiting will be like when you throw up after having eaten something bad or due to indigestion. When the thrown out liquid is foamy and whitish, you have kapha vitiation.

If you throw up thick and stinky liquid, you suffer from amadosha, which means that you have accumulated inside your stomach parts of undigested food. Patients of amadosha sometimes vomit out some blood. Normally such patients have a very hard stomach and often suffer from troubles related to digestion. Emesis cures amadosha but one should also consult an appropriate physician.

Vamana aftercare: After vamana, you should take rest for about two hours. Drink a tea made from basil, fennel and cardamom (see the recipes given under antara dhauti) or simply drink warm cardamom water. You can have something light to eat after about two hours. For meals, eat porridge, semolina halwa, vegetable soup or soupy khichari (refer to my book *Ayurvedic Food Culture and Recipes* for details of preparation). For the next two days, take light meals and do not do any strenuous work.

On the third or fourth day after vamana, do the oil saturation massage to prepare yourself for the next cleansing practice. Eat simple but health-promoting meals like vegetable soups, fruit salads and warm and unctuous main courses. Use health-promoting spices like curcuma, cumin, fennel, ginger, dill, coriander and fenugreek. Do not use chillies during this period. You need to rebuild your strength before purgation with health-promoting food and appropriate rest.

2. Virechana or Purgation

Virechana, the second of the seven cleansing practices is easier to do as compared to vamana or the voluntary vomiting. Virechana is voluntary purgation and it is induced by taking an herbal mixture. This practice cleans the liver and other digestive glands, and throws out excessive heat from the body through stool.

Virechana is the major treatment for curing pitta imbalance.

Choice and dose of the purgative: In each country and each region, people know various plant purgatives which they take to cure constipation. For virechana, however, you need a strong herbal purgative. It could be a mixture of several plants. Powder of Sanaye (*Cassia augustifolia*) leaves is a very good purgative for purification. Take about 1 teaspoon of this powder with warm water before going to bed.

Alternatively, the pulp of amaltas (*Cassia fistula*) can be taken. Take out the pulp from about 12-13 cm (about 5 inches) of the bean stock. Beans are between 30 cm (1 foot) to 60 cm (2 feet) long. Boil the pulp in a little water. Mash it properly and filter it through a strainer. Drink it at night before going to bed.

Reaction: Purgatives are taken in the evening before going to bed. They work inside you during the night and, depending on your state of health, you may have stomach ache or flatus before you get loose motions. The reaction time naturally varies from one individual to another. Some of you may feel a strong urge to go to the toilet during the early hours of the morning; others will need some time after getting up and have to drink something before the reaction begins. It is not important when the purging begins. If you do not purge properly and you have only one or two motions, repeat the process with a higher dose.

Results: Purgation works on the agni or the digestive fire of the body and throws out also the other imbalances from the digestive tract. Some of you may release a lot of wind which is a sign of vata vikriti. Whitish stool along with mucous indicates kapha imbalance. Pitta disturbance is cured by throwing out excessive heat from the body and those of you who suffer from too much sweating or other similar symptoms, will have a feeling of relief after purgation.

After purgation: Take the same precautions as after vamana: some rest and drink plentiful. Take only light meals for two days and on the third or fourth day, repeat the oil saturation massage. Take normal and healthy meals to rebuild your strength and prepare yourself for enemas.

Basti or Enemas

Enemas are the third and fourth of the seven cleansing practices. There are two kinds of enemas—unctuous and non-unctuous. The unctuous enema (anuvasana basti) is applied with fat and the non-unctuous enema (asthapana basti) is with special herbal decoction. Enemas are of tremendous importance for cleaning the body. Charaka has said in Siddhistana (VII, 64):

> **Enema, though done in a localised part of the body- the colon, draws up impurities from the soles of the feet to the head by its power as the sun situated in the sky evaporates the humidity from the earth.**

Enemas are not only used for routine purification, they also form a part of the Ayurvedic therapeutics. Enemas with various decoctions are applied for curing various ailments.

Enemas are recommended for those who are stiffened, contracted, lame, afflicted with dislocation and in whose extremities aggravated vata is moving. Enema is prescribed in distension of the abdomen due to the presence of gas, knotted faeces, colic pain, aversion to food and other such disorders of the gastrointestinal tract. Enema is beneficial for those women who do not conceive... due to complications caused by vata.

Enemas are the major treatment to re-establish the equilibrium of vata.

Enema apparatus: For the application of enemas, you require an enema apparatus, which is easily available from the medical stores or drug stores. It has a pot of about 2 litre capacity with an outlet. A rubber tube of about 150 cm (5 feet) is attached to this outlet and the end of this tube has a catheter with a nozzle and a tap to control the outflow of the liquid. The enema pot has a small hole or a hook so that you can hang it up (Figure 73). You need some place where you can hang the apparatus and a bench or a table below it to lie down upon.

3. Anuvasana Basti or Unctuous enema

A week after the purgation, apply the unctuous enema. The quantity of the liquid inserted for unctuous enema is 250 ml (1 ¼ cup).

Recipe for the unctuous enema liquid:

Milk	160 ml (4/5 cup)
Sesame or olive oil	30 ml or 2 tablespoons
Ghee	30 ml or two tablespoons
Honey	30 ml or two tablespoons

Mix the first three ingredients, heat a little and whip well. Then add honey into this mixture and mix well.

Just before the application of the enema, heat this mixture to about 35^0 C. Do not heat it above that temperature. Feel the temperature with your finger. It should be a little more than the body temperature or like a warm bath or shower. Honey is antagonist to heat and that is why it is important not to heat it too much. If by mistake you overheat this mixture, throw it away and make a new one. Overheated honey produces toxins in the body.

Time for enema: The best time for enema is about two hours after breakfast or lunch. Do not do enema on an empty stomach or immediately after evacuation.

Enema posture: It is important to practice the posture for enema beforehand. Lie down on your left side with your left leg folded and right leg straight (Figure 74). Let yourself completely loose and breathe deeply. Make sure that you do not stiffen any part of your body and you are not anxious about inserting the enema liquid inside you for rinsing your colon. Think that it is like rinsing your mouth every morning with water.

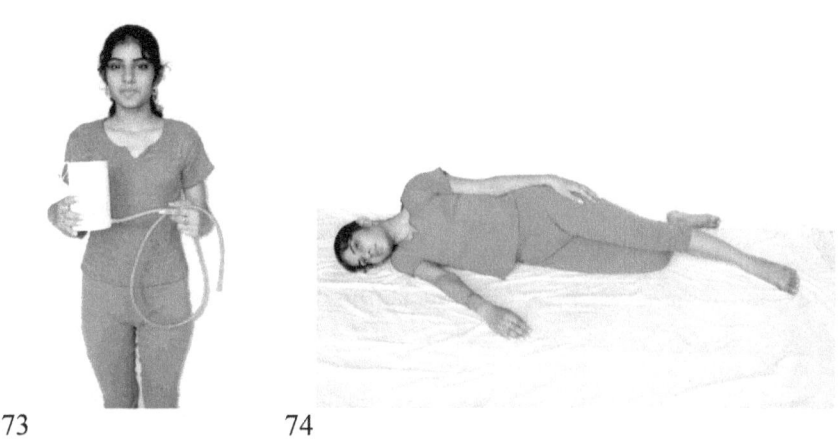

73   74

Inserting the unctuous enema: Put the warm mixture into the enema pot, open the nozzle and take out the air from the tube. Wait until the first few drops of the liquid come out and then close the nozzle. Keep a teaspoon of ghee or coconut oil close to you. Hang the pot at an appropriate height above the bench or table you have prepared for lying down. Now make the posture for enema as described above. Insert your finger in some ghee or oil and smear your anus with it to facilitate the insertion of the nozzle. Insert the nozzle into your anus and open the tap. When all the liquid has gone inside you, take the nozzle out and keep lying down in the same posture for a few minutes. Get up slowly, and walk around for a minute. After that you sit or lie down again. Avoid any fast movements. The longer the liquid stays inside you, the better it is. Try and forget that you have inserted something inside you. Go to the toilet when you have a strong urge for it.

After the unctuous enema: It is quite possible that a part of the liquid stays inside you for a day, which is very good. If it comes out too quickly or practically all of it at once, it means that the liquid did not have enough time to work inside the colon. If this happens, try and apply the enema once again. Repeat some mantra to attain a state of relaxation. Those who are suffering from vata vitiation, are nervous and those who lead a hectic life-style often have this inability to hold the enema liquid. Normally, after the purvakarma with several massages, fomentation and fat drinking, even these people are quite relaxed. Another aspect is that some persons are scared of inserting something into the anus. If this is the case, try and convince yourself that it is not an odd thing you are going to do, you are simply using a different way of cleaning yourself.

Follow the same diet as suggested for the first two cleansing practices. You need to relax for a day after applying the next enema.

4. Non-Unctuous Enema

The non-unctuous enema should be applied one day after the unctuous enema. The procedure is the same except that now you use about 1 Litre (5 cups) of special herbal decoction. For a one-year-old child, the dose of enema liquid is 40 ml and with each added year, it increases 40 ml (about 1 fluid ounce) up to 12 years of age. After the age of 12, increase the dose by 80 ml (2 fluid ounces) per year up to the age of 18. That makes a dose of 960 ml (nearly 5 cups) for an adult. After 70 years of age, the dose should be reduced to 800 ml (4 cups).

Various decoctions for non-unctuous enema

Depending upon your prakriti or particular state of vikriti, you can take a number of decoctions for this enema. However, there are few plants or the combination of plants that help create equilibrium and they will be helpful for all kinds of prakriti.

Triphala decoction for equilibrium of three doshas

Triphala is made with three fruits—Amala (*Emblica officinalis*), Harada (*Terminalia chebula*) and Baheda (*Terminalia bellirica)* in equal quantities.

Dried fruits are weighed after taking out their seeds and they are powdered. Triphala can be bought in a pharmacy but take care to see the date. Herbal products, particularly when powdered, expire within a year or at least their qualities deteriorate. You will find more details on Triphala in Chapter 9.

Add 2 tablespoons of triphala powder into 1¼ litre (6 cups) water and bring it to boil. Put the lid on and cook it on very low heat for about 15 minutes. Let it lie like this for another 15 minutes. You can filter it and reheat it to an appropriate temperature before the application of the enema. The temperature should be the same as you use for taking a bath or a shower.

Triphala is not always available in Western countries. If you cannot get it, use other herbs that have a similar effect to create equilibrium. The two famous plants that help re-establish the harmony are Camomile and Saint John's Wort. Use the same method to make the decoction. Powder the herb and make the decoction with the same amount as for triphala.

Decoctions for vata

For treating vata imbalance, you use one or more of the following herbs; anise, fennel, coriander, verbena, fenugreek (methi) or liquorice. Use the same method as described above for making decoctions.

Decoction for pitta and vata-pitta

Make a mixture of anise, fennel, coriander and liquorice in equal quantity for preparing this decoction. These herbs are good for both vata and pitta vitiation.

Decoctions for kapha

In this case use thyme or ajwain. Alternatively take one tablespoon of powdered pomegranate peels and one tablespoon of powdered liquorice, fennel or anise.

Decoction for kapha-pitta

Use coriander or a mixture of anise and cumin to make a decoction. Prepare the decoction in the same way by powdering the herbs as described above.

Decoction for vata-kapha

For this decoction, you powder four big cardamoms and boil them in water for 15 minutes. Alternatively, you can take one tablespoon of kalonji or half a nutmeg

Note: If you are not sure about your specific condition, use triphala or the other two balancing herbs mentioned above.

Application of non-unctuous enema: This enema is applied in a similar manner as the unctuous enema. The difference here is that you are inserting a liquid that is lighter in consistency but four times more in volume. For best results, you should be in a relaxed and peaceful state. You should be able to hold the liquid inside you and do not get an immediate urge to purge it out. The other precautions and instructions are the same as described for the unctuous enema.

5. Nasya or Purification of the Head Region

Nasya is fifth of the seven saptakarma practices. Nasya is the Sanskrit word for nasal passage which is considered to be the gateway to the head region. In addition to the sense of smell, it is also a way to reach other senses—sight, taste and hearing. To purify the head region, medication is applied through the nasal passage, a procedure called Nasyakarma meaning 'action through the nasal passage'. This practice is meant for revitalising the four senses, the nervous system and for insuring an appropriate intake of prana.

The classical Nasyakarma is difficult to do without the help of a physician. I have discovered a simpler way of doing it through inhalation of medicated vapours or herbal smoke from some specific herbs. However, the effects of my methods are milder as compared to the classical nasyakarma and should therefore be applied more often.

Inhalation with medicated vapours

For this practice, you need two things—the inhalation equipment and inhalation oil.

Inhalation device: The electric inhalation apparatus with thermostat can be bought and in some countries it is also called—'Face Sauna'. If you are unable to get it, the inhalations can be done in a big ceramic cup. Heat the cup with boiling water, throw out that water and add more boiling water into it. The vapours can last in it for about five minutes. The third alternative is to buy a small thermos and put a funnel on the top. Lastly, you may use a small pot of boiling water on an electric stove and inhale directly from there. A gas stove is not recommended. In fact, this last way is the simplest and the most effective.

Inhalation oil: Use a mixture of various etheric oils like eucalyptus, citronella, anise, clove along with menthol crystal and camphor. Usually these mixtures are sold as medication for a cold. Such oils are also used in commercial balms like Tiger balm or Ayurvedic balms like Amritanjan balm. Thus, you can also use a little of one of these balms in the boiling water.

Inhalation: The room where you inhale should not have any air draft. Put a scarf on your head to keep it warm. If you are inhaling from a ceramic cup, cover it with a thick paper so that the vapours are not wasted.

When your inhalation apparatus is ready and you have boiling water in it, add some drops of inhalation oil or about ¼ teaspoon of the above-mentioned balms. Put your nose close to the vapours and take deep breaths alternatively from mouth and nose (Figure 75). Try to keep the vapours inside you for a few seconds as you have learnt in the pranayama practice. This may make you cough and spit several times and you may have to blow your nose. Do not swallow the saliva as to spit it out is a part of purification. You will realise that gradually your nasal passage is cleared and you are able to breathe in the strong vapours with ease and more profoundly. The next step is to close the right nasal passage with your finger and inhale 4–5 times only from the left side (Figure 76). Repeat the same from the right nasal passage after closing the left side.

For the third step, inhale deeply, close both your nasal passages and the mouth and push the vapours with great force as if you want to send them to all parts in the head region (Figure 77). You will feel the effect of the vapours all over and also in your ears. Let the vapours out when you cannot hold them anymore. Repeat 4-5 times.

If you are using an inhalation device without a thermostat, it is quite possible that you do not have any more vapours for the next step. You have to take another cup of boiling water with fresh oil in it. Even with a thermostat, you may have to add fresh oil into the water so that the vapours are strong enough for the next step.

Inhale deeply, close your nose with your fingers and also shut your mouth, and then lean your head backwards (Figure 78). While you are leaning backwards, also tilt your head sideways. Hold the vapours as long as you can and then let them out. Repeat this step also five times.

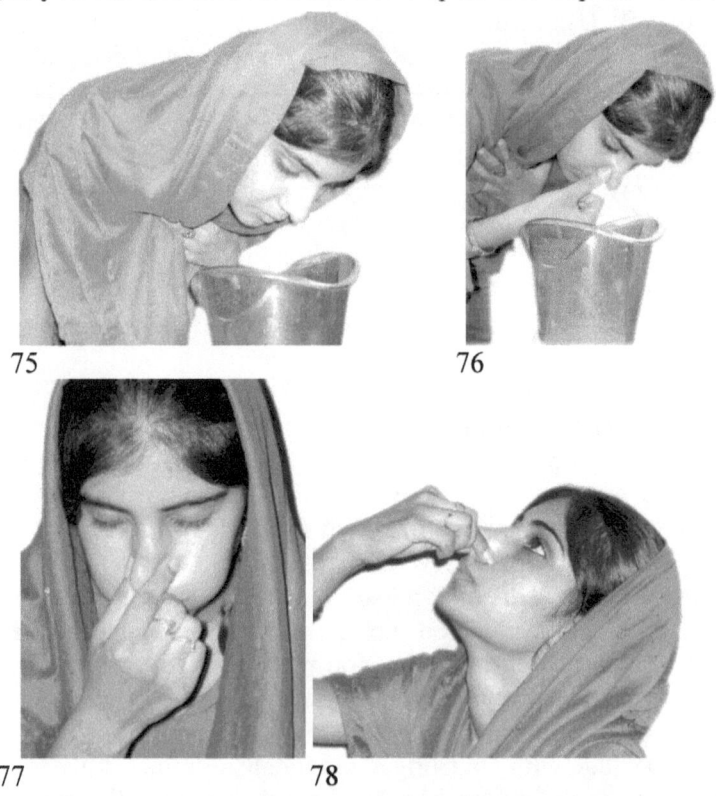

75   76

77   78

Time and frequency: The inhalation should be done three times during the half yearly cleansing practices. It does not require much time; ideally you do it before going to bed on weekdays.

6. Raktashodhana or Blood Purification

Blood purification is the sixth of the seven purification practices and it comprises of taking a mixture of some specific substances for detoxifying the blood. Through imbalance of humours, wrong food, chemical sprays, fertilisers, etc., we constantly accumulate toxins in our blood. This is why we have to detoxify our blood at regular intervals. Special purification substances gradually work on the body and throw out the toxins through body excretions like stool, urine and sweat.

Note: Blood purification is also a remedy for allergies, skin eruptions, pimples, acne, excessive heat and body odour.

Blood purifying substances: Certain plants are capable of detoxifying the blood and some of them are also used in our cuisine. The most common examples are fenugreek (methi), basil (tulsi), ajwain and bitter gourd (karela). Traditionally, in India, people also use neem fruit (nimboli) as vegetable because it is one of the important blood purifiers and not as bitter as the rest of the products from the neem tree. This fruit grows during the monsoon season and its regular intake keeps away the frequently occurring monsoon ailments like fevers (including malaria), boils or other waterborne infections.I give below a simple and balanced recipe for the blood purifier. Blood purifying substances have a dominant bitter rasa and therefore need to be balanced with other rasas.

Blood purifier

Kalonji	10 gm (½ ounce)
Cress seeds (chansoor)	10 gm (½ ounce)
Ajwain	10 gm (½ ounce)
Fenugreek seeds (methi)	10 gm (½ ounce)
Cassia absus (chaksu)	10 gm (½ ounce)
Basil leaves (Tulsi)	10 gm (½ ounce)
Neem leaves	10 gm (½ ounce)
Liquorice (mullathi)	30 gm (1½ ounce)

Dry all ingredients and powder them with the help of a small spice grinder or a coffee grinder. Mix the powder properly and pass it through a fine strainer. If there are big pieces left on the strainer, grind them again. Pass through the strainer again and throw away the left-overs. Mix the powder well with a spoon and keep it in a tightly closed jar.

Intake: Take half a teaspoon of the above preparation daily for 15 days. Put the powder in your mouth and swallow it with water. It is bitter and may be unpleasant for some of you. You can eat something sweet afterwards to get rid of the bitter taste in your mouth.

If you are suffering from excessive heat or skin eruptions, too much sweating, body odour or other effects of pitta vitiation, you may continue to take the blood purifier for 30 days.

Timings: Take the blood purifier after the enemas and continue for 15 days. The best time to take the blood purifier is in the evening before going to bed.

Effect of the blood purifier: The blood purifier may give you mild diarrhoea from time to time. It is a part of the purification process, so you need not worry.

7. Bastishodhana or Purification of the Urinary Tract (Diuresis)

This is last of the seven cleaning practices and it consists of taking strong diuretic products in order to flush out and clean the urinary system completely. For this practice, you need half a day free.

Diuretic substances: There are many diuretic teas or herbal mixtures that can be used for this purpose. A pinch of barley salt (java kshar) followed by a lot of liquid does the cleansing very effectively. In the West, many herbal teas which are sold for curing bladder infections also serve this purpose. In India, a few glasses of sugarcane juice can do this purification very effectively. To reduce the diuretic effect of the sugarcane, the juice makers generally add ginger in this juice. But for diuretic effect, you should take sugarcane juice without ginger. Fresh pineapple juice can also serve the same purpose.

Intake of diuretic substances: Take the diuretic substance either one hour after breakfast or two hours after lunch. If you are taking barley salt, dissolve a pinch of it (about ¼ of a teaspoon) in a glass of water and drink it. Keep drinking something afterwards. You can drink some fresh fruit juice or herbal tea with anise, fennel, verbena, thyme or ajwain. Do not drink ginger tea, as ginger is anti-diuretic. You can also drink a light normal black tea. In hot weather, you can drink sherbets or fresh lemon juice in water with a little candy sugar. In any case, for about two hours, keep drinking something every 15 minutes. You will be going to the toilet very often and the strong effect will last for about four hours and then gradually diminish.

If you are doing the purification with sugarcane or pineapple juice, first drink half a litre, then twice a quarter litre one and two hours later. You will keep having to go to the toilet. After about two more hours, drink cardamom water or plain water. You can also drink herbal teas as has been mentioned above.

After diuresis: The effect of diuretic substances goes away slowly. It is quite possible that for the following 24 hours you have the urge to urine more often than usual. It is essential to take fluids. Have soups or other warm and fluid things the following two days.

The diuretic substances work within the water system of our body. They are cold in nature. Therefore, it is very important that you keep yourself warm after diuresis. Do not take rice, cold milk, bananas or other substances that are also cold in their Ayurvedic nature (see Table 6). Take appropriate rest at least that evening. Do not take a cold shower after diuresis or expose yourself to a draft.

Complete Saptakarma Schedule

Although I already have suggested above individual schedules for each practice, it seems appropriate at this point to sum up all Saptakarma activities. Please ensure that you leave an appropriate space of time between each practice during which you saturate your body with oil.

I have given above a schedule of 10 days for purvakarma and I will continue from thereafter.

Day 12 Vamana (emesis or voluntary vomiting)

Day 15 Oil saturation massage

Day 19 Virechana (purgation)

Day 22   Oil saturation massage
Day 25   Unctuous enema
Day 26   Non-unctuous enema
Day 32   Diuresis
Days 11, 14 and 17   Inhalation
Days 28 through 42   Blood Purification

Note: It is a suggested schedule, you can alter it to suit your work schedule but take care that you follow the basic pattern.

PASHCHATKARMA: CARE AFTER CLEANING PRACTICES

I have described above the post-purification care in each case and now I will give some more details on pashchatkarma.

Light, warm and liquid food: Purification practices are tiring for the body and one looses a large quantity of fluid in this process. With the purification practices, we are renewing our three fundamental energies. After throwing out the *malas* or impurities, we have to rebuild our energy gradually. After each purification practice, we need to take food that assimilates easily in the body. Vegetable soups with ajwain and cumin, thin khichari, porridge, semolina halwa, steamed vegetables, baked or boiled potatoes are good examples. Vegetables that fall in the category of balanced food like carrots, pumpkin, courgette and turnip should be used. Pepper, chilli and other spices with a pungent taste should not be used. Use of butter or ghee should be done during this food preparation. Use cumin, fennel, cardamom and ajwain to spice the food. Except after the diuresis, you can also eat rice boiled in water. Take salt and sugar in moderate quantities and avoid sour things. Do not eat raw vegetables and salads. Fruits like papaya, banana, sweet grapes, pomegranate, sweet apples can be taken but avoid fruits with sour rasa. Eat a moderate quantity of food.

Intake of fluids: You lose lots of fluid through the various cleansing and preparatory practices and therefore it is essential that you drink a lot during this time. Warm cardamom water is highly recommended. Water is the greatest purifier. Besides, cardamom water helps re-establish the equilibrium. Do not take any aerated drinks or pre-pressed and preserved juices. Freshly pressed juices of sweet fruits and different kinds of herbal teas with mild rasas are recommended.

Sufficient rest and sleep: After the cleansing practices, some rest is required as the process of inner cleansing is very tiring. Besides, the cleansing process exerts the internal organs of the body; therefore you need a calm and peaceful atmosphere and appropriate rest. For example, if you have applied an enema, it is better to rest at home for several hours. It is quite possible that some of the liquid may suddenly come out many hours later. To recover from the fatigue of inner cleansing, you need a good night's rest also. Avoid going to bed late. This is the time to rejuvenate your energy, take as much rest as you can.

No hectic activity for two days: Do not over-exert yourself, do not carry heavy things or run or do any kind of hectic exercise for at least two days after the application of cleansing practices. Try and reduce stress by repeating PSAUV several times a day. When we are under stress, our internal organs also stiffen. This should be avoided. Pay attention and let yourself loose. With these precautions you will be able to take full advantage of the cleaning practices.

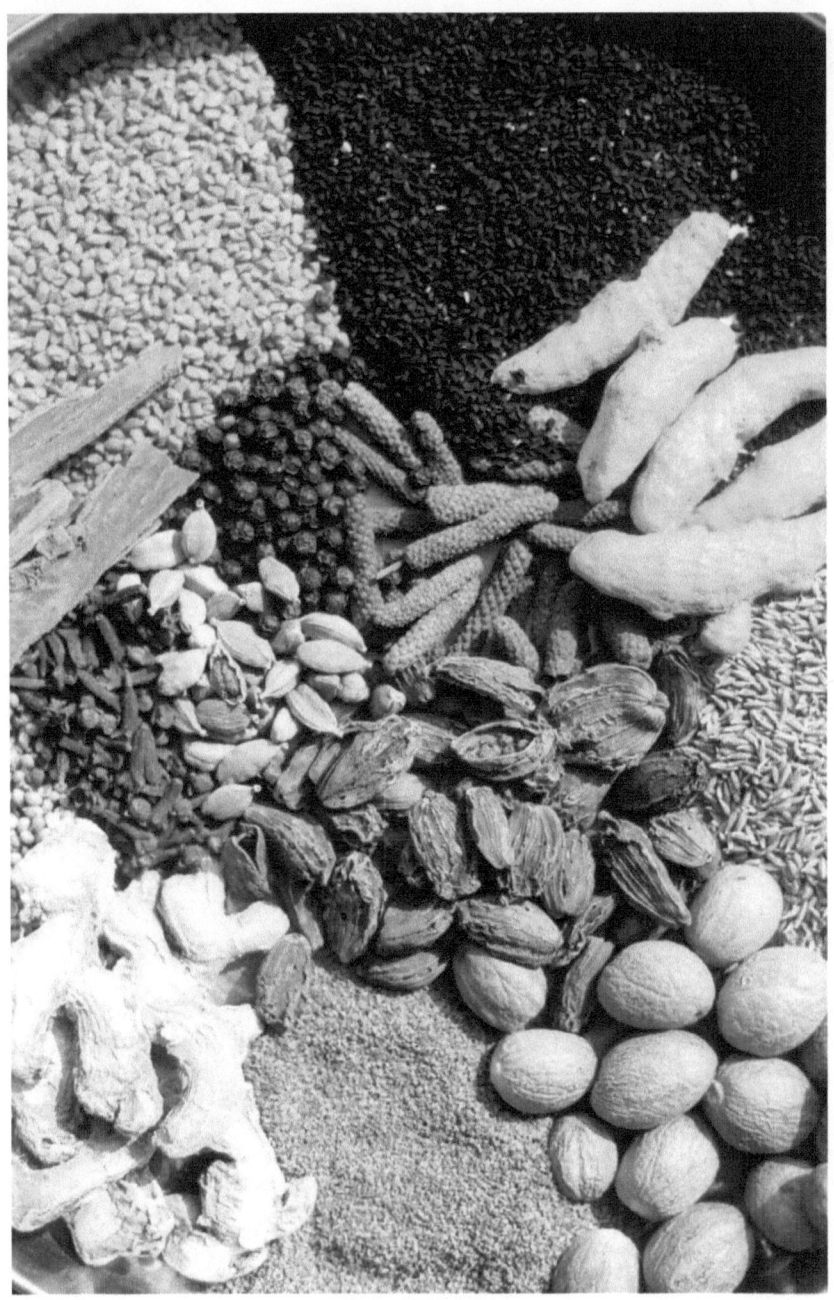

Chapter 7

Remedies and Rasayanas

I will deal with three themes in this Chapter. Firstly, you should become familiar with the remedies you need to revert back from the state of vikriti to prakriti. Secondly, I am giving you a few remedies for treating some very common minor disorders. Thirdly, I am giving several recipes for rasayanas. You should take rasayanas or health promoting products regularly so that your ojas (immunity and vitality) remain high. Rasayanas enhance the quality of life, meaning that you can live up to your optimum energy level. They are also preventive against ailments as they strengthen the immune system.

Remedies for Vikriti

You have already looked at several methods to diagnose prakriti and are now able to distinguish between the state of health and non-health. The aim of Ayurvedic practice is to help nature re-establish itself. When you feel unwell due to one reason or another and find yourself in a state of vikriti, you should know the remedies to return to prakriti or the state of well-being. If there are any disorders building up in the body, they should be nipped in the bud. You should make a multidimensional effort to revert back to prakriti and thus, help nature to maintain its order and bless you with health. With multidimensional efforts like nutrition, yoga, herbal remedies, sattvic thoughts, appropriate rest and so on, you can re-establish your harmony and regain your usual strength and vitality rapidly.

Vata vikriti

Symptoms: Your dominant vital energy is liable to vikriti due to change of weather or other factors related to that. For example if you have vata prakriti, the windy weather will affect you more. Travelling, walking too much, a hectic lifestyle, dry and cold food, preserved or pre-cooked (basa) foods are the factors which will lead to vata vitiation. You may feel the effect of this vitiation through diverse symptoms like constipation, dry throat, stiffness in the body and at times restless sleep. It does not however mean that the only vikriti you can have is of your dominating dosha. We will discuss that later. But first let us see how you should manage your vata vikriti.

Remedies: It is important to look into the factors that cause the vata vitiation in your particular case, especially if it happens often. Some persons may get this vitiation due to certain foods like some kind of lentils or beans, over-ripe peas or a certain kind of bread with yeast. It is extremely important to eradicate these factors that divert your prakriti to vikriti often. Other than that, take the following measures:

- Drinking hot water is a remedial measure for vata vitiation.
- Do the oil saturation massage with warm oil as has been explained earlier in Chapter 4 in the weekly programme.
- Take warm bath, dry fomentation and appropriate rest.
- Eat warm and unctuous food predominant in sweet and sour rasas. Avoid pungent, astringent and bitter substances.
- Take only hot foods and drinks and avoid all cold foods and drinks.
- Recommended foods are milk, banana, papaya, citrus fruits, carrots, turnips, fenugreek (methi), kalonji, cumin, fennel, dill, cardamom and ginger.
- To cure vata vitiation, take herbal tea with basil and liquorice. Add 4-5 basil leaves and a half-teaspoon of powdered liquorice in half litre water. Bring it to boil and let it cook for about five minutes on a low fire with the lid on. Put off the fire and let it stay like this for a few minutes. Filter and drink it.
- If your vata vitiation is caused due to an exposure to cold and you have stiffness and body ache, boil 6-7 crushed cardamoms and 7-8 leaves of basil in half litre water for five minutes. Keep the preparation covered and cook on a low fire. Drink it in two doses. You may add some candy sugar in it for taste.
  If you are suffering from fatigue due to vata, take an herbal tea with big cardamom, clove and cinnamon. Crush one big cardamom, three cloves and a small piece of cinnamon and boil these in half litre water. Let it cook covered on low fire for about five

minutes. You may add some candy sugar into it to sweeten. This preparation can also be taken as normal tea or chai with the addition of black tea and milk into it.

- Ajwain or thyme tea is also good to alleviate vata vitiation. Dose for ajwain or Thyme is half a teaspoon in half a litre of water. Make the tea as described above.

- Ginger, basil and cardamom tea is very effective in vitiated vata. Crush about 3 cubic centimetres of ginger, 5 basil leaves and 3 cardamoms. Add all this in half a litre of water and make the tea in a similar manner as has been described above. In case you do not have fresh ginger, replace it with half teaspoon of powdered ginger. Add some candy sugar in the end to make the spicy taste of the ginger milder.

- For treating vata imbalance, take one clove of garlic daily, crush it and add ¼ of a teaspoon of ghee and swallow it. Do not drink anything cold after taking this preparation.

- Crush one teaspoon each of kalonji and cumin along with two teaspoons of candy sugar. Split this into six doses and take three times a day for two days. If you think that you are still not completely cured from the symptoms of vata vitiation, repeat this for another few days.

- If your vata vitiation is too frequent and intense, you should take the treatment for 15 days or more with chaturbeej churan (powder of four seeds). Powder the following four different kinds of seeds in equal quantity: fenugreek, ajwain, cress and kalonji. Take half a teaspoon of this powder 3 to 4 times a day.

Note: *Cress seeds are easily available everywhere. Ask for Garden Cress seeds. In Europe, the leaves of cress are eaten as a salad. In India, its cultivation is done to feed horses. It is called Chandarshoor in Sanskrit, Chansoor and Halim are some other North Indian names. In Tamil it is called Alivirai, in Telegu- Adeli, in Kanara- Allibeej.*

Pitta vikriti

Symptoms: One or more of the following symptoms indicate that you have an imbalance of this energy: excessive heat in the body, skin ruptures, herpes or pimples or indigestion, sour taste in the mouth, too much hunger or thirst or too much sweat, yellow coloured urine and body odour, bouts of anger

Remedies: Avoid all those factors that vitiate pitta. Do not take alcoholic beverage; eat simple food that is not too much spiced or salted. Avoid chillies, pepper or anything else that gives a burning sensation. Avoid being in the sun and in the afternoon heat. Thus, eradicate all those factors that bring more heat to your body.

Take the following measures to bring the vitiated pitta to equilibrium:

- Drink plenty of water, cold milk and cooling sherbets like brahmi or sandalwood.
- Take a cold bath and apply cooling ointments like sandalwood paste, ghee or coconut oil on your body. If you have burning sensation in a specific part of the body, you may apply sandalwood paste only on that specific part of the body.
- Take mud treatment. Yellow and fine variety of earth is used for this purpose. It is also called 'healing earth' or 'Multani mitti' in India. Make a thin paste with this earth by adding water and do an anointing with it on all over your body (*lepa*). Leave it for about half an hour and wash it off. This treatment will also make your skin smooth.
- Take foods that are dominant in sweet, bitter and astringent rasas. Suggested foods are rice, masoor dal, spinach, carrots, cabbage, pumpkin, courgette, aubergine, bitter gourd, dates, bananas, sweet apples and grapes, papaya, cold milk, ghee, fresh cheese (paneer), fennel, clove, coriander and liquorice.
- Take herbal teas like wormwood, neem, coriander and liquorice. Take extremely bitter substances only in a very moderate quantity. Use a few leaves of neem or wormwood and mix them with some ajwain to make the tea. The reason for this is that exclusively bitter rasa may cure your vitiated pitta but in turn may vitiate your vata. Equilibrium of drugs is important in Ayurvedic pharmacology.
- Take a teaspoon of juice of bitter gourd (*karela*) two times a day to pacify the excessive heat in the body.

Masoor dal soup with ghee is an effective dietary measure to cure vitiated pitta. The recipe is given below.

Masoor Dal Soup

Masoor dal	100gm or ½ cup
Fennel	¼ teaspoon
Curcuma	¼ teaspoon
Salt	to taste
Ghee	3 teaspoons
Coriander leaves (chopped)	1 tablespoon*

Clean and wash the dal a few times and let it soak for about 15 minutes. Boil ½ litre (2 ½ cups) of water and put the dal into it after draining out the water. Add spices and salt and cook on a low fire with a lid on for about half an hour. Stir from time to time. At the end if the water is soaked and the preparation is thick, add more water to make it soupy and boil it after adding the water. Add the chopped coriander leaves in the end and add ghee before serving.

If coriander leaves are not available, add crushed coriander seeds along with other spices.

Kapha vikriti

Symptoms: The symptoms of kapha vikriti are: a sweet taste in mouth, too much salivation, foamy urine, sticky stool and desire to sleep a lot. You may get a feeling of heaviness in your body and may feel drowsy, lazy and passive.

Remedies: It is important to avoid all those factors that lead to kapha vitiation. Oily, fatty, salty and heavy to digest foods should be avoided. Sedentary habits and lack of exercise vitiate this dosha further and therefore you should force yourself to be active and go out for a walk or other activities.

To reverse the state of kapha vikriti into your natural state or prakriti, take the following measures:

- Use spices like ginger, garlic, dill seeds, kalonji, fenugreek and mustard seeds.
- Take always freshly prepared hot food.
- Hot bath and vapour bath are very effective in curing kapha vikriti.

- Force yourself to do physical exercise and go for walks.
- Make an effort to keep awake (less sleep).
- Make an effort to go out, meet people rather than sitting alone and feeling drowsy.
- Avoid watching too much television.
- Suggested foods are Soya beans, potatoes, cress salad, tomatoes, cauli-flower, peaches, plumbs, citrus fruits and honey. Ghee should be avoided and cooking should be done in moderate quantity of sesame or olive oil. Sugar and products containing sugar should not be taken. To sweeten tea or coffee, use candy sugar.
- Take a clove of garlic everyday with some honey.
- Take herbal tea with ginger, cardamom, pepper and basil.

I have described above the remedies for vikriti of the three principal doshas. As I said before, normally the dominant dosha of the prakriti is more vulnerable to be vitiated. Nevertheless, depending upon the circumstances, your environment, your activities and your mental state, any other vital energy may also get an imbalance. That is why it is essential to do the daily observations for your diagnosis. Imagine that you have vata or pitta prakriti and generally you see that you get vitiation of these two doshas from time to time. However, one time you suddenly notice sweet taste in your mouth, heaviness in your body and feel drowsy during the daytime. You may notice that you have sticky stool, foamy urine and excessive salivation. If you have these symptoms or some of them, they indicate the vitiation of kapha. Try and reason out why did this happen. It may turn out that the intake of cold milk in winter, eating too many sweet things like rice, bread and sugar-containing preparations had led to kapha vikriti. Therefore it is essential to do your daily diagnosis carefully. Take the steps described above for curing vitiated kapha.

Vikriti in Excess

I have described above several remedial measures for getting back to the state of prakriti from vikriti. It is possible that sometimes these measures may give you relief but not completely and you may again revert back to the state of vikriti. It would mean that your state of vikriti is quite intense and you have to take major measures. Saptakarma purifies the whole body, throws out all the imbalances and re-establishes the balance of the three principal energies of the body—the vata, pitta and kapha. As I have stated earlier, the reason to purify the body with saptakarma practices every six months is never to let the disharmony or the state of vikriti to stay long in the body.

It is possible that sometimes you are unable to do saptakarma practices for a while but you require taking some measures to revert back to the state of prakriti. Always remember the major cure for each of the doshas:

- Enemas are to cure vata vitiation
- Purgation is to cure pitta vitiation
- Emesis or voluntary vomiting is to cure kapha vitiation

In an intense state of vikriti, you can use these cleansing practices individually. For example if you are repeatedly getting symptoms of vata vitiation, you may apply enemas. But take care that before applying enemas, you prepare your body with oil saturation massage and fomentation. If you have been suffering from constipation, take a mild purgative one or two days before applying enemas. The reason for this is that if there is a substantial amount of excrements left in your intestines, they may be pushed back with the enema fluid.

In case of pitta vitiation, take purgation and you will get immediate relief. For example, if you have frequent indigestion or too much sweating and body odour, you will find that after doing a good purgation, these symptoms will disappear or get milder. You can repeat purgation after about two weeks if your symptoms do not completely disappear.

In case of kapha vitiation, emesis or voluntary vomiting has to be done. If you frequently get the symptoms of kapha vitiation, I suggest that you do the yogic practice of jaladhauti once or twice a week.

In all the cases of vitiation, it is important to follow the other instructions about nutrition, sleep and lifestyle in general for maintaining the equilibrium of the three basic energies. If you are unable to get back to the state of prakriti from vikriti despite all your efforts, you should see a competent physician. Sometime there is a disorder or an infection in the body and the vitiation is repeatedly caused because of that. When we have an outer attack or a malfunction of an organism, the body is struggling against it and during that time various symptoms like fatigue or vikriti of the three energies are apparent.

Finding the Lost Equilibrium

It is possible that two or all the three energies of the body are imbalanced at the same time. Sometimes you may feel fatigued and find that your energy level is low. This state may also confuse you and you find yourself unable to diagnose yourself. In this case, you need to take something more special to re-establish the equilibrium. Saptakarma practices are known to uproot the imbalances and the disorders created due to them (see Chapter 6). There are also certain substances that throw out the imbalance from the body and re-establish the harmony. It is considered that the drugs do not uproot the disorders; they just cut the offshoots of the tree that is in the form of imbalance. Triphala is a very well known drug for this purpose and needs explanation.

Triphala: Triphala means three fruits. This drug is a mixture of three fruits in equal quantities. These three fruits are Amala (*Emblica officinalis*), Harada (*Terminalia chebula*) and Baheda (*Terminalia bellirica*). These fruits have big seeds and for making triphala, they are weighed in dried form without their seeds and are powdered. Pass this powder through a fine strainer and discard the leftovers. Mix well and store in a tightly closed jar and keep in a cool place.

Triphala can be also bought readymade as most Ayurvedic companies make it. It is one of the basic drugs of Ayurveda. Pansaris (shopkeepers with herbal materials) also keep it in the ready form. If you buy the packaged product, make sure you look at the date. It should not be more than six months old. The other day, somebody brought a bottle of triphala to me in Delhi that was packed 4 years ago. In such cases, the medicinal properties of the plants disappear. The pansaris who sell a lot to the vaidyas (Ayurvedic physicians) generally have fresh preparations. Pass it through a fine strainer nevertheless and use only the fine powder.

How to use triphala: Since triphala is a well-known Ayurvedic drug, sometimes people do not use it properly or have misconceptions about it. Many think that it is simply a drug to cure constipation. It is important that you know all the qualities of this drug and its correct usage for various remedies.

All the three plants used in triphala are health-promoting and are rasayanas. Therefore, triphala is used in many rasayanas in Ayurveda.

Triphala re-establishes the balance in the body and therefore different persons will have different reactions to it. The reactions are according to the imbalance that prevails. Triphala purifies the body. Triphala is used in many Ayurvedic drugs to create a balance in them.

- If you wish to use triphala for re-establishing the equilibrium of the doshas, take it in the following manner: Soak one to two teaspoons of the powder in about 200 ml (1 cup) hot water in a china or glass pot and stir well. Keep over-night. Next morning, warm it a little and filter it. Drink on an empty stomach.
- Triphala is also taken to lose weight and for that it should be taken in a similar manner.
- For enhancing vision, triphala is mixed with honey and made into a paste. Keep this paste for 2-3 days and stir it several times. Take a teaspoon of it every night before going to bed.
- Triphala can also be mixed with one third of its quantity of honey, ghee and liquorice each and taken as rasayana for promoting vision.

As said above, triphala is a rasayana and it is added in several rasayana preparations. But you may take triphala in the above manner in honey or with ghee, etc. in case of fatigue and anaemia.

I do not recommend that you take triphala as such in dry form or in the form of tablets as some companies have started making it in recent years. Though convenient for consumption, it is not meant to be taken in this form. Some people just put the powder in their mouth and swallow it with water. If you are taking triphala for losing weight, take it in the above manner (soaked in water) along with other precautions described for Ayurvedic nutrition, like never filling your stomach more than two thirds, never eating before the previous meal is digested and so on. The role of triphala in this case is to create a balance between mala (excrements) and rasa (food that is absorbed in the body). Proper elimination of mala and a balance and harmony of the three energies of the body will help you to shed weight. Besides that, when you reduce your diet in quantity, triphala with its rejuvenating qualities will help you to feel active and healthy. For more details on this theme, see my book, *Losing Weight with Yoga and Ayurveda.*

Effect of triphala: Tiphala is a rejuvenating dietary supplement. As said before, it is a valuable drug which re-establishes the equilibrium of doshas and therefore different people react differently to it depending upon the imbalance they have. In healthy persons, triphala enhances stool and urine after its intake and thus purifies the system.

In case of **vata vitiation**, in addition to enhanced stool, there would also be wind release for the first few days and you may feel a churning sensation in your stomach.

In case of **pitta vitiation**, you will also have large quantities of stool but it would be thin and watery. That means that the system is throwing out excess of heat.

In case of **kapha vitiation**, you may feel sick after drinking triphala in the morning and some of you may feel like vomiting. Your body is getting rid of an imbalance of kapha and throwing out excessive phlegm.

Do not get discouraged by these symptoms after taking triphala. The reason I give all this in detail is that many people take triphala after having read about its wonderful qualities and are frightened by the symptoms that follow the intake. They think and many tell me that triphala does not suit them. But reading all these pages on Ayurvedic practice, you must have understood that in Ayurveda, the symptoms of any imbalance and disorder are not suppressed like in allopathy. They are dealt with and are uprooted. The functions and properties of each energy are very precise and the effect of various drugs on them is very specific. Triphala works on the body in a similar manner as the major saptakarma practices to re-create the equilibrium. Recall that the major cure for kapha imbalance is emesis or voluntary vomiting. For re-establishing the balance of pitta, purgation is the major method. Vata is brought to harmony by enemas. Triphala acts in a similar manner.

If you have imbalance of more than one dosha, you may have various effects over a period of time. I suggest that you take triphala for 10 days from time to time. If you want to take it as a rasayana, triphala is mixed with other things and a recipe for this is described later in this chapter.

Saint John's Wort: This is a European herb that creates balance of doshas. It is interesting that like triphala, this herb is used to cure diverse ailments and is added in different remedies in traditional German and Swiss herbal medicines. Some opponents of traditional and herbal medicine criticise such drugs by saying that it is unscientific to use one plant or one drug to cure diverse ailments. However, in the light of Ayurvedic wisdom and looking at it from a holistic point of view, many troubles arise because of a fundamental imbalance in the body. There are products in nature which are capable of re-establishing this balance. You have noticed in the list of nutrients that there is also a category of food products, which is balanced. Thus, everything that brings balance of the three energies of the body cures all those symptoms of vikriti which arise due to that specific imbalance. These plants or combinations of plants simply help your body to restore itself to the state of well-being; that is from the state of vikriti to prakriti.

Doses and intake: Saint John's Wort is a small plant that can also be grown in pots but needs a temperate climate. Its leaves and fruits are used for medicinal purposes. It is also sold in the form of tea bags in Europe. In case of imbalance, drink its tea twice a day. One teaspoon of the herb or a tea bag makes one cup (about 200 ml) of tea. This should be considered as one dose. Pour boiling water on it and brew it for 10 minutes. You may add some candy sugar to sweeten it.

Camomile: This is another European plant for bringing equilibrium of humours. Its leaves and flowers are also used for medicinal purposes. The dose is the same as described for Saint John's Wort. Camomile tea is also used to wash sore eyes or to cure a cold, fever, etc. If you are taking Camomile or Saint John's Wort as a remedy, you should take it 2 to 3 times a day. Make a cup of tea (about 200 ml) from one tea-spoon or a tea bag each time.

Other Methods of Regaining Equilibrium

I understand that when you have lost the equilibrium of the three ener-gies of the body and have various symptoms relating to it, you may be quite confused at times. Therefore it is important that you should know diverse methods to treat yourself. Nutrition is a powerful medium to treat our ailments as well as to make us sick. In the present context, I want to suggest that if you have several problems and are confused about your state of health or you feel that all your three doshas are in vikriti, go on a special diet of very simple food with little fat. You will find below some recipes for that diet. With this kind of food for a few days, many of your problems related to digestion will vanish on their own and you will get a good feeling in your body. With some of these problems gone, it will be easier for you to analyse yourself and treat. Change of environment is another way that is helpful to regain balance and harmony. Change of place not only changes air, water and climate, but it is mentally refreshing also.

Nutrition measures: Here are some ideas for a very simple diet to purify your system. Take this food for a week and if you feel better, integrate some of its recipes in your routine menu. The diet contains more nutrients from the balanced foods (see Table 6).

Breakfast

Cook 2-3 grated carrots with a little water and some cardamom in them for about 15 minutes. Add into this preparation a little candy sugar if you want it sweeter than the carrots usually are. Add ½ to 1 teaspoon of ghee in the end. Those of you who cannot digest ghee may add a glass of milk instead. But if you use milk, cook for another 5 minutes.

Alternatively, have plain yoghurt with some rice. Cook rice in double its quantity of water after having soaked it for 15 minutes. Cook it covered on a very low fire. Cooking time for Basmati rice is about 8-9 minutes: Let it lie covered for another 3 minutes after cooking. Separately, whip the yoghurt and add a little salt, pepper and ½ a teaspoon of roasted and ground cumin. This quantity of the cumin is meant for one person. Cumin can be roasted briefly on a hot pan and then crushed in a small mortar.

Meals: Eat fresh and warm meals and do not eat meat or eggs while on this special diet. Have only small and light meals. Do not take late dinners, make sure that you have it at least two hours before going to bed. One should do this anyway, but be especially careful when you are unwell. Avoid bread with yeast or other pre-prepared food. I give below some special recipes for dinner.

1. Carrot soup is highly recommended for dinner. Cook about three carrots with one potato in ¾ litre of water for about 20 minutes on low fire, with the lid on. After 10 minutes, add to it ½ teaspoon each of curcuma (turmeric) and cumin. Add also ¼ teaspoon each of fennel, ajwain, dill seeds, coriander and salt and pepper according to taste. After everything is cooked, purée it in a mixer. Add some butter or ghee before serving.

2. Balanced vegetables like courgette, pumpkin, carrots are always good to eat. You may add other vegetables to your menu but avoid vegetables like cauliflower, cabbage or others of this family. They are generally hard to digest. Use always fresh ginger along with vegetables and add spices like cardamom, ajwain, cumin, dill seeds, coriander, clove and fennel. It is easy to prepare a spice mixture for your diet: mix all these spices in equal quantity except clove which should be taken in half the quantity.

3. You can add rice or roast potatoes to your menu. Eat only freshly prepared bread.

4. For dessert, eat fruits like papaya, sweet apples, sweet mangoes and pomegranate. Mixed fruit salad is highly recommended.

5. Those of you with weak digestion should avoid salads and raw vegetables. Use herbs like coriander, dill, basil and others to garnish the vegetables and soups.

Do not eat anything between meals. Avoid taking alcoholic beverages during this period. Drink your morning hot water and take hot water with cardamom at other times also when you are thirsty. In case you get a feeling of heaviness or bloating, take lemon-ajwain after the meals (see later in this chapter for the recipe). If you have a lack of appetite, take lemon-ajwain half an hour before the meals along with a little fresh ginger.

Change of Environment

Many a times, a change of environment is very helpful in re-establishing the equilibrium of the body and it gives a sense of well-being almost immediately. There are several factors in the environment—water and air being the most important. I have an interesting little story to tell in this context. The climate of forests and mountains is vata dominating and some people living in these areas may experience constant fatigue due to vata vitiation. Such was the case for an acquaintance who lived in the Black Forest (Germany). He was constantly complaining of various aches and pains or related troubles. He lived in Delhi for two years and once he told me that he had never felt so good in his life as he felt in Delhi. People of Delhi who are constantly grumbling about the air and noise pollution and the ailments arising from them were utterly surprised from this statement. But this person was able to be free from his vata imbalance because of the midland and hot climate of Delhi as compared to the vata dominant cold climate of the mountains and forest of his homeland. This story shows how powerful the effect of climate can be.

If you are suffering from vikriti, think of taking some holiday at a restful place where the climate is entirely different. The effect of any particular climate is very strong on you if you do not live and eat properly accordingly. For example, if you are in the mountains or live in places which receive air from the mountains and where often dry winds are blowing (called Föhn in German), you are prone to vata vikriti. But if you eat warm food with garlic, ginger, fenugreek and ajwain, not expose yourself to wind directly and take a hot bath every day, your vital energy will not be disturbed. However, if instead you eat dry and cold food and often have those vegetables and grains that enhance vata, you will certainly suffer from vikriti of this dosha. If you will not pay attention and leave this vitiation unattended, it will gradually enhance and give rise to one or more vata ailments. Pay attention and if there is vitiation, a holiday in midlands or on the seashore will do you good.

If you live near the sea or another such place with very humid climate, you may get kapha vikriti if you eat sweet and fatty food and do not do enough physical exercise. In that case, take a holiday in the mountains or midlands for a change of climate. In a hot climate and specially if you have to work outside and are exposed to the sun, you can accumulate too much heat and get pitta imbalance. The cool air of the mountains and forest areas will do you good. Go near a water source but not where it is hot.

There are also temporary effects of all kinds of weather on us and some people may get vikriti due to it. Take appropriate care, diagnose yourself properly everyday and take an appropriate action immediately. Normally the effect of weather like windy days or a sudden wave of heat goes away by itself with the change of weather. For example, in the month of *Phagun* (mid March to mid April), there is windy weather in northwest India. This is vata weather. Everybody has to be careful and especially those with vata prakriti. We should always be alert and prepare ourselves for the change of weather. It is called Ritucharya (living according to the season) in Ayurvedic terminology. In essence, Ayurveda is the science that teaches us to follow the rhythm of nature and join the flow of the cosmos with appropriate way of life.

Vikriti and External Attacks

The state of vikriti makes us vulnerable to external attacks. It lowers the ojas (immunity and vitality) and thus we become liable to external infections like bacteria, virus, etc. If we are in a state of equilibrium and are taking rasayanas and balanced nutrition, then our ojas are high and the body fights back the attacks of external infections proficiently. In fact, many of you may observe that when you have high energy and vitality and your body is in a state of equilibrium, you are saved from common cold or similar attacks even when they are in epidemic proportions. Thus, maintaining the state of prakriti and enhancing the ojas by taking rasayanas are essential to save one from external attacks.

Remedies for Some Common Ailments

The field of Ayurvedic remedies is extremely broad and complicated, and an exhaustive presentation would be beyond the scope of this handbook. For our purpose it will be sufficient to look at a few selected home remedies. In fact, this book is meant principally to describe the routine practices of Ayurveda in some detail and it is a workbook or do-it-yourself book. Besides that, if I write about remedies, you will also require explanations of various ingredients and diverse preparation modes. I have described several remedies and preparation modes in my book: *Ayurveda, A way of Life*. Thus, in this book, I will keep this theme limited to a few home remedies.

Common Cold

I give below several measures which can be taken simultaneously to fight back the common cold.

A Remedy with Chickpea Flour or Besan

This is a very common home remedy and is very easy to prepare.

Chickpea flour (besan)	2 tablespoons
Ghee	2 teaspoons
Water	200 ml (1 cup)
Candy sugar	2 teaspoons or according to taste

Fry besan in ghee on a low heat, and stir constantly. After about a minute, add water and stir well so that the besan does not form lumps. Add also sugar and cook for another minute.

Drink this preparation while it is hot. Do not expose yourself to a draft or cold afterwards. Preferably lie down for a while and cover yourself. You may sweat after drinking this.

Dose: The above quantity is for one dose. Depending upon how bad your cold is, take the preparation between two to four times a day.

Inhalation

Inhalation with medicated vapours is extremely important in the cold season. It prevents the blocking of the nasal passages and sinus with phlegm. The method and importance of head purification or nasya with diverse modes of inhalations has been described earlier in saptakarma practices. It is exactly this practice you need to do to cure common cold. If you are suffering from cold, take the inhalations twice a day until it is cured. If you have problems with sinus, you continue the inhalation practices for several days until all the blocked phlegm gradually comes out.

Basil, Cardamom, Ginger and Pepper Tea

This tea with the four above-cited ingredients can be taken for pleasure or to cure the common cold and fever. The difference between food and medicine is that in case of the latter, the doses and their frequency are prescribed. For pleasure, this tea is made milder whereas it should be stronger for a remedy.

Ginger (fresh and chopped)	1 tablespoon
or	
Dried ginger	½ teaspoon
Black pepper	5-6 grain
Basil leaves	about 10
Cardamom	5
Candy sugar	according to taste
Water	600 ml (3 cups)

Crush the ingredients and put them in water. Bring to boil and cook for about 15 minutes, covered, on a low heat. You can add candy sugar in the end. Split it into three portions and take a dose every 4 hours. Do not expose yourself to cold or draft after drinking this tea.
Note: This tea is for both cold and fever as it is also analgesic. It is to treat the fever that is due to vata or due to an exposure to cold or is accompanying an attack of cold and cough. Do not take this tea if your fever is due to exposure to the sun or heat. Then you need a preparation with bitter rasas.

157

Fevers

As stated above, in Ayurveda, various types of fevers are treated differently. But there are remedies which are predominant in several rasas and are used to cure all kinds of fevers. Giloye (Guduchi in Sanskrit and *Tinospora cardifolia* in Latin) is one such example. Giloye is also a rasayana. It is a very tough and fast growing wild plant and can be grown in a pot at home. I have narrated in the next Chapter a story of my personal experience and wonder healing with this plant.

Giloye Preparation

The giloye stem is used for medicinal purpose. Take out about 15 cm (6 inches) long fresh stem. Dried stem can also be used. In that case, powder it and take half a teaspoon for a dose. The powder can be gulped down with water. In case of fresh stem, cut it into small pieces and boil in about 200 ml (1 cup) of water until the pieces are soft. Mash them with a mixer or just with hand to get the pulp out. Filter it and cook the extract for another 2-3 minutes after adding 2 teaspoons of candy sugar. Drink this preparation and if the fever still persists, take another dose after 6 to 8 hours.

Preparation with Neem, and Chirayata

Neem (dried leaves)	10 gm
Chirayata	10 gm
Giloye (dried)	10 gm
Ajwain	20 gm
Pepper	5 gm
Fennel	10 gm

Clean, dry and powder all the ingredients. Pass through a fine strainer to obtain a powder. Store in a clean and dry bottle.

Dose: Take half teaspoon of this powder every four hours in case of fever. This mixture is quite bitter. Put it in your mouth and swallow with water. You can eat something sweet afterwards.

Note: Bitter rasa can vitiate vata. That is the reason why in this preparation, ajwain, pepper and fennel are added to make it a balanced preparation.

Cough

A very simple home-remedy for coughs is made with honey, pepper, basil and juice from fresh ginger.

Ginger	2-3 cubic centimetre (1 cubic inch)
Black pepper	5 grains
Basil leaves	5
Honey	1 tablespoon

Crush ginger in a mortar until the juice comes out. In this juice, crush pepper and basil leaves until you get a paste. Add honey into this paste and eat it. This quantity is for one dose. Take 2 to three times a day depending upon the gravity of your cough. It is essential to take a dose before going to bed.

Chronic cough

If your cough is persistent and does not go away with the above remedy, you require something stronger. Sitopaladi is an extremely effective traditional Ayurvedic medicine. It is sold in the market but it is also fairly easy to make. It can be mixed with honey and can be preserved for a long time. Most of you are familiar with the contents used in this recipe except one and that is vanshalochan (or tavaseer in North-west India). Vanshalochan literally means 'eye of the bamboo'. It is an extract from the bamboo plant (*Bambusa arundinacea*) and it looks like an eye on the upper part of the plant. Due to the non-availability of the natural product, the synthetic equivalent is sold in the market and is equally effective. It contains various silicon salts.

The classical formulation for making sitopaladi is described below.

Sitopaladi

Candy sugar	50 gm
Vanshalochan	25gm
Long pepper or pippali	12 gm
Cardamom	6 gm
Cinnamon	3 gm

Take the cardamom out of their pods and grind all the ingredients in a small spice or coffee grinder. Pass the powder through a very fine strainer to obtain a fine powder. Mix well and add honey to make a paste. Usually, you require three times the quantity of honey to make a paste. But depending upon the type of honey, you may need a little more or less.

Dose: Take four times a day, about one third of a teaspoon each time. Give half the dose to children. Always take a dose before going to bed. Do not drink water or anything cold after taking Sitopaladi.

If you have chronic cough or cold and you feel that your head region gets blocked with phlegm, mix Sitopaladi powder in ghee instead of honey. Take it for 3-4 weeks or until completely cured. Take four times a day in the beginning and reduce the dose gradually to twice daily.

Loss of Appetite, Indigestion and Alcohol Hangover

Loss of appetite is a problem especially amongst children. Childhood is predominantly kapha and children of kapha prakriti are more vulnerable to this problem than that of the other two types. Loss of appetite occurs due to excessive heat or kapha vitiation. Imbalance of kapha suppresses the digestive fire.

Ginger, ajwain and lemon are some household products used as a remedy for loss of appetite.

- Cut thin slices of ginger and sprinkle some rock salt (Sendha namak) on it. Put some lemon juice on the preparation. Eat some of these pieces half an hour before your meals.
- Lemon juice with ajwain and rock salt is also very effective for

this purpose. In fact, this preparation is also very good to treat a feeling of heaviness after meals. It is also good to get rid of a hangover from alcohol.

- For loss of appetite, take ½ teaspoon of ajwain with half teaspoon of lemon juice and a pinch of rock salt half an hour before your meals.
- For indigestion or alcohol hangover, take the same dose after meals or after alcohol. Repeat after two hours if needed.
- If you feel sick or you find that the food you had is not digested or assimilated, take the above dose every two hours until you feel better.
- In case of stomach ache, take lemon-ajwain with hot water. Put ½ teaspoon of lemon-ajwain in your mouth and swallow it with hot water. You can also chew ajwain and then drink hot water.

The above preparation is known as lemon-ajwain or nimbu-ajwain and is available in the market. You can also make it at home. If you are travelling, you should always have some of it with you.

Lemon-Ajwain

Ajwain	100 gm (½ cup)
Lemon juice	50 ml (¼ cup)
Rock salt	1 tablespoon

Put the ajwain in water. The stones and earth will go down to the bottom whereas the ajwain seeds will float on the top. Take out the floating ajwain from water with a strainer and spread it on a clean cloth to dry. Spread the dried ajwain on a plate and add half the lemon juice and all the salt. Ajwain should be drenched with lemon juice. After a few hours, it will absorb some of the juice and some water contents will evaporate. Add the rest of the juice and mix it with a wooden spoon. This preparation will dry in one or two days depending upon the weather. When it is absolutely dry, store it in a clean and dry jar. Take half a teaspoon when needed. Either chew it and eat gradually or swallow it with some warm water.

Stomach Acidity

Stomach acidity is another frequent problem many people suffer from but it is easy to cure with some home remedies.

161

Stomach acidity can be cured with specific nutritional measures and a regular practice of jaladhauti. Nutritional measures to bring the balance of the doshas have been described earlier in this Chapter.

Do not sit or lie down after meals. Go for a slow walk or just move around. You can sit in rock posture after a meal. A similar position is shown in FEEP (Figure 22).

If you are suffering from acidity, do not eat spicy, sour or pungent food. Avoid anything sour, also fruit. Balance sour rasa with salty, sweet and bitter rasas.

Perhaps everybody knows that a glass of cold and sweetened milk after meals helps alleviate acidity. But take care that the milk you take is of good quality.

Clove-Raisin Remedy for Acidity

Cloves	10 gm (½ ounce)
Dried raisins	30 gm (½ ounce)

Powder the cloves and mix them with raisins. Make a paste of these two in a mortar. If it is dry and does not turn into paste, you may add a little honey. Make tablets of a size of fresh green pea by rolling a little piece of this paste between your palms. These tablets can be stored in the refrigerator for about a week.

Dose: Take one to two tablets after meals. Chew very slowly and let the contents go inside you gradually.

Treatment for Minor Skin Problems, Allergies and Pimples

I discuss these problems together because basically they all are related to blood and you treat them with blood purifier. The recipe and dose for the blood purifier has been described in the last chapter. Do the treatment for a month and take a special simple diet described earlier in this chapter.

If you have a persistent problem with skin eruptions, pimples and other minor allergies, do a long-term Curcuma cure. Take a teaspoon of powdered curcuma (turmeric or Haldi in Hindi) everyday for several months. The simple method to consume this dose of curcuma is to make a glass of curcuma milk which is not only remedial for allergies and purifies the blood, but it is also strength promoting.

Curcuma milk is very easy to make and it also tastes very good.

Curcuma Milk

Curcuma	1 teaspoon
Ghee	1 teaspoon
Milk	150 ml (¾ cup)
Candy sugar	1 to 2 teaspoons or according to taste

Melt ghee in a pan and add curcuma, stir-fry it on a very low heat for about half a minute. Add sugar and stir for another half a minute. Be careful to keep the heat very low during this time. Add milk, stir, increase the heat and bring it to boil. Some thick contents of the curcuma powder will settle at the bottom of your cup. Drink while it is hot.

Caution: Beware of the curcuma stains. They normally do not go away with soap. They become lighter with an exposure to sunshine.

Fatigue

Fatigue is not an ailment by itself but if unattended, it can give rise to diverse ailments and disorders.

Take appropriate rest and try to build up a peaceful atmosphere around you. Remember the fundamental mantra of Ayurveda- **the first priority of life is life itself.** There is a saying in my part of the country- 'human beings come to an end—work never comes to an end'. Stop saying that 'there is so much to do, I cannot rest'. This kind of attitude is an invitation to get big ailments related to heart, liver, blood and brain. Try and do those things which give you pleasure and relaxation. If you are confused and cannot decide what gives you pleasure or you are too tired to decide, go to some faraway place for a holiday. If your immediate surroundings, like your family fatigues you, go away alone for a short while. Also make sure that you take Rasayana V (described below) twice a day.

Rasayanas or the Strength Promoting Special Preparations

We observe around us that when there are infections like cold, cough, influenza and other viral or bacterial infections, many people become victims. Many a time, especially in big cities, they turn into epidemics. Nevertheless, there are some persons who have better resistance to infections and they are saved from the attacks. We also observe that there are times that we have better resistance to infections than at other times. When we are tired or have a stressful mental state, we fall prey to external attacks.

Ayurveda recommends taking health-promoting products so that our level of resistance to ailments remains high and we can enhance our vitality. Immunity and vitality together are termed as 'ojas' in Ayurveda. Enhanced ojas helps us to fight back the effect of aging and give us a better quality of life and longevity. Let me sum up below the definition of a rasayana.

A rasayana is that substance or a group of substances that have several rasas in concentration. The intake of rasayanas brings equilibrium to the body and supplies vital dietary elements or rasas. It also enhances digestion and assimilation. Rasayanas rejuvenate the body by increasing ojas (immunity and vitality) and thus help fight back the effect of ageing and provide longevity.

Rasayanas are a very significant part of Ayurvedic wisdom. One of the eight branches of Ayurveda is devoted to rejuvenation and longevity. Along with other practices described in this book, it is also necessary that you take rasayanas regularly to enhance your ojas and have a radiant look. I give you some recipes of rasayanas which are easy to make.

Rasayana I: Garlic as Rasayana

Many substances in nature are rasayanas. A strong rasayana that all of you are familiar with is garlic. Garlic has five out of six rasas. It does not have the sour rasa and has the other five rasas described in Ayurveda (sweet, saline, pungent, bitter and astringent). Since garlic is very strong, it should be taken in low doses for the purpose of rasayana. Depending on a person's prakriti, it should be taken in different manners.

Vata dominated persons should take it crushed with little ghee.

Pitta dominated persons should crush it with some candy sugar and take it with cold water.

Kapha prakriti persons should crush it and add a little honey to it.

Dose: The doses of garlic as rasayana should be according to your capacity to digest. Begin with only one small clove of garlic and increase it to two cloves if you are able to digest it properly. It is better to take it regularly in small doses than irregularly and excessively.

The smell of garlic is offensive to some people and therefore to reduce it, chew cardamoms and drink plenty of water. Garlic smells from the mouth, sweat and urine. Take a decoction of coriander to suppress the garlic smell. Powder the coriander and make it like herbal tea.

Garlic rasayana can also be made by preserving it in honey and persons of diverse prakriti can take it. Garlic as such is heavy to digest. However, this preparation makes it easier to digest and milder in its smell.

Garlic	100 gm (4 ounces)
Honey	300 gm (3/4 lb)
Cloves (spice)	10 gm (½ ounce)

Prepare garlic by peeling it off. Spread the garlic cloves on a flat surface and let them dry for a few hours. Take a glass jar of ½ litre (2 ½ cup) capacity and put garlic cloves into it. Pour the honey on the top and stir everything together with a spoon. Garlic floats in the honey and you need to push it down so that all the cloves of the garlic are well smeared. Add the cloves (the spice cloves, not cloves of garlic) in the jar and stir all the contents well. Close the jar well and keep it in a cupboard. Open it every day to stir the contents or do so by shaking the jar. The garlic 'matures' in about 10 days and can then be eaten.

Dose: Begin with one clove a day along with one spice clove. You can increase the dose up to three cloves a day depending upon your digestive capacity. But always take one spice clove with the garlic cloves. Take before going to bed.

Rasayana II: Saffron

Saffron is a rasayana and an aphrodisiac that promotes sexual energy and vigour. It can be taken in a simple manner with milk. If you do not drink milk, dissolve it in a few spoons of hot water and then take it. For saffron recipes with milk and almonds, you may consult my book *Ayurveda Food Culture and Recipes*. Saffron can also be consumed in rice or in desserts.

The Latin name of the plant that gives saffron is *Crocus sativus*. What we know as saffron that is used as spice and medicine is the stamina of its flowers. Saffron looks like tiny fibrous substance with bright orange colour.

Quality of saffron: You have to be very careful to get good quality saffron without any adulteration. Saffron is grown in Kashmir and it is also imported from Spain and Southern France. It is said that the Kashmiri saffron is the best quality for medicinal use. Be careful as there is lot of adulteration in saffron. The perfume of pure saffron is very strong.

Dose: Daily dose of saffron as rasayana is 100 mg. You can split a one gm packing into 10 doses.

Rasayana III: A Simple Preparation Against Fatigue

This preparation is simple and the ingredients described here are present in an Ayurvedic kitchen.

Anti-Fatigue Remedy

Cumin	2 tablespoons
Fennel	1 tablespoon
Kalonji	1 tablespoon
Dried ginger (powdered)	1 tablespoon
Cardamom (seeds)	1 tablespoon

Grind all the ingredients after cleaning and drying them. Pass the powder through a strainer to obtain a fine powder. You can also use cheesecloth for this purpose. You can consume the powder in three different manners described below to get rid of fatigue and to revitalise yourself.

Different modes of intake and doses

i.   Take half a teaspoon of the powder twice a day.

ii.   If you wish, add 3 tablespoons of powdered candy sugar into this preparation to make it more palatable. Increase the dose a little in this case.

iii. To make a fine preparation from these ingredients, add them in 400 ml of rose water. Leave the contents for 24 hours at room temperature and shake the bottle from time to time. Add 3 tablespoons of powdered candy sugar and shake well to dissolve it. Keep it in the refrigerator. Some contents will dissolve and others will settle at the bottom. Take 2 tablespoons each in the morning and in the evening from the liquid. Do not shake the bottle and let the undissolved contents stay at the bottom. When you have taken all the liquid, discard the remaining contents.

Rasayana IV: Brain Rejuvenating Nuts in Honey

This is recommended for children as well as for people who have to do brainwork. It can be taken every day, about 10 minutes before breakfast.

Brain Rasayana

Cashew nuts	200 gm (½ pound)
Pumpkin seeds	100 gm (¼ pound)
Almonds (peeled)	100 gm (¼ pound)
Fennel	50 gm (2 ounces)
Black pepper	25 gm (1 ounce)
Cardamom	25 gm
Honey	1 Kg

Take a jar of 2 kg and put honey in it. Add cashew nuts, pumpkin seeds and almonds. Peel off the cardamom and powder them along with pepper and fennel. Add all the spices into the jar. Stir the contents well and close the jar tightly. Let everything 'ripen' for about a week. Shake the jar from time to time so that the contents are well immersed.

This preparation tastes very good as the nuts in honey acquire a very special taste. It can also be served as dessert.

Dose: Daily dose is one to two tablespoons before breakfast. You can also take at any other time of the day but two hours after taking your meals.

Rasayana V: Anti-Fatigue Rejuvenating Rasayana

This is a comprehensive rasayana you can use every day to enhance your physical and mental capabilities and to increase your immunity and vitality.

Ingredients:

Brahmi	50 gm	Fennel	50 gm
Shankhpushpi	50 gm	Basil (Tulsi leaves)	25 gm
Triphala*	100 gm	Neem leaves	25 gm
Trikuta**	100 gm	Ajwain	50 gm
Cardamom	25 gm	Giloye	25 gm
Big cardamom	25 gm	Ashvagandha	25 gm
Clove	25 gm	Fenugreek (Methi)	25 gm
Cinnamon	25 gm	Coriander (Dhaniya)	50 gm
Dill seeds	25 gm	Liquorice (Mullethi)	50 gm

Clean and dry everything. Take the cardamoms out of their pods. Powder everything with a coffee grinder or a spice grinder. Large substances like liquorice or dried ginger should be made into small pieces with a stone or iron mortar so that they do not break the knife of the grinder. Pass this powder through a fine strainer and crush the rough pieces again. Pass them through the strainer and discard the contents which are still rough. Mix the powder with honey and stir well. Normally, you will need three times more the volume of honey than the volume of powder. The powder soaks the honey and it becomes like a paste.

Dose: Depending on your body weight, take from 1 to 1½ teaspoon everyday. In case of fatigue, take a spoonful and lie down for about half an hour. Drink something hot afterwards. You will feel the effect immediately.

*Triphala has been already described earlier in this chapter.
**Trikuta is a mixture of black pepper, long pepper (pippali) and dried ginger in equal quantities.

Note: If you cannot get some of the ingredients, you may leave them out. Your rasayana will still be effective.

Preservation: After mixing the contents with honey, the preparation can be kept for a long time. Keep in tightly closed jars and preserve in a cool and dry place. For everyday use, keep a smaller quantity in a little container.

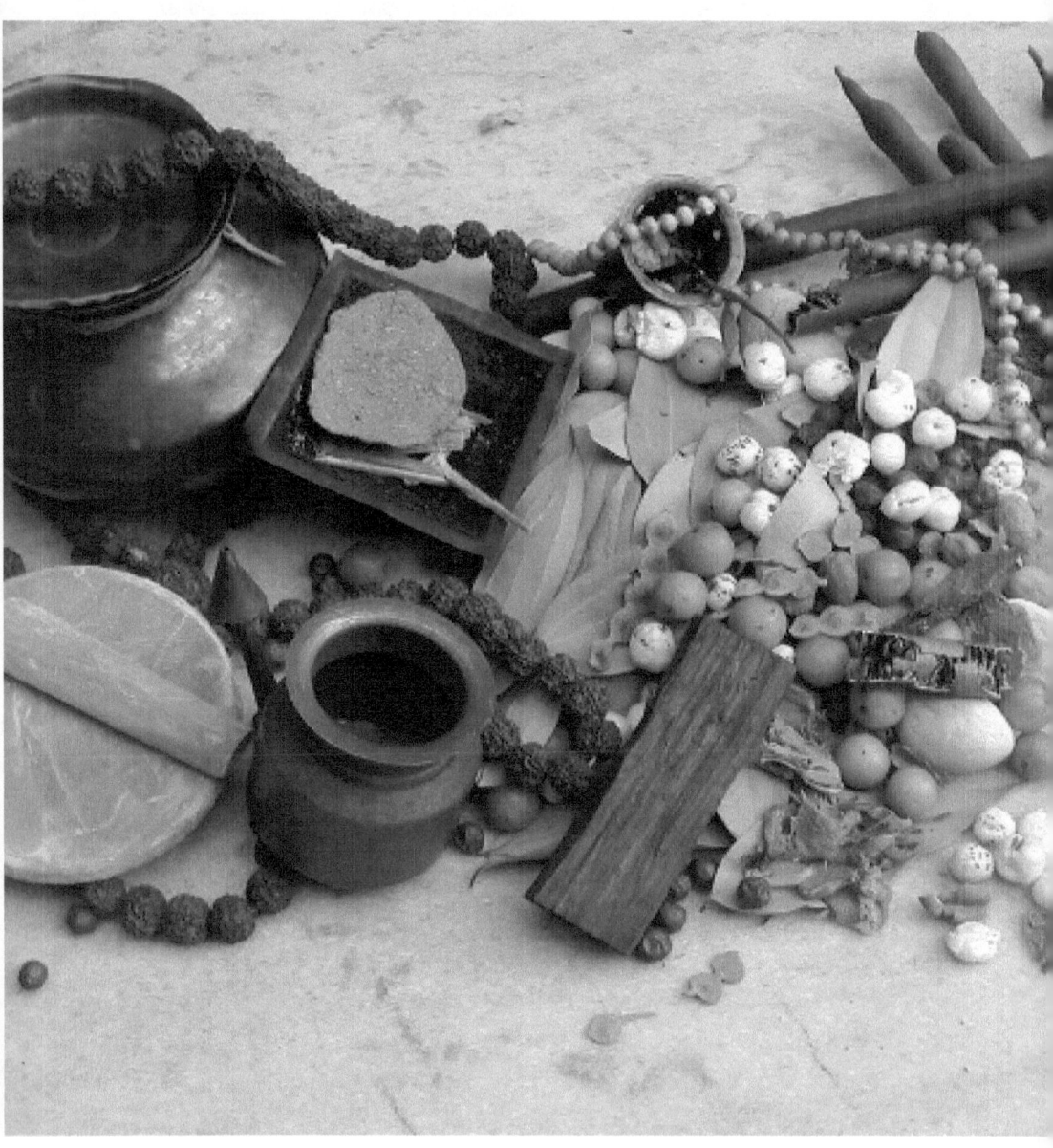

Chapter 8

Some Other Aspects of Ayurvedic Life

In 1987, I returned from Germany to live in India for six months in order to do research on the use of Ayurvedic methods to promote health and prevent ailments. Although our masses use the traditional methods of medicine, Ayurveda with a foreign popularity stamp on it had not yet touched the urbanised folks who had lost their traditional values. Later, I came to India to stay longer to write my first and basic book on Ayurveda (*Ayurveda, A Way of Life*) and I recall that I could not impress many in Delhi with my ideas. In fact, the book first appeared in German and other European languages and then in America. It took me many years to have it published in India. Meanwhile, in the mid-nineties, Ayurveda had acquired popularity in the Western nations, and Sri Lankans and Keralites made it into a popular business for foreigners. Our Indian elite refreshed the old memories with a long 'a' at the end of the 'Ayurvedaa'.

Vata, pitta, kapha, abhiyanga, panchakarma and shirodhara have become popular terms of health care abroad. This evolution of our thousands of years old health care and medical system was delightful but unfortunately remained one-sided. Many involved in the spread of Ayurveda were not properly educated in Shashtriya (scriptural) tradition and thus missed out the other two most important aspects of Ayurvedic prevention and therapy—the psychological and spiritual. In the first Chapter of this book, I have given several citations from Atharvaveda, the first source book on Ayurveda, to highlight these aspects. I cite below what Charaka said 2600 years ago (Sutrasthana, VIII, 27):

One should not postpone things at the time of action nor should one take up anything without examining it. One should not be submissive to his sense organs nor should one have an unstable mental state. One should not over-burden the sense organs, nor should one be dilatory. One should not act under the emotions of anger and exhilaration. One should not live under continuous grief. One should not feel exhilarated in success and depressed in failure. One should always keep in mind one's constitution. One should be confident of the effect of the cause and as such should always initiate the cause. One should not assume that now nothing could be done. One should not give up courage and nor should one remember one's scandals.

My idea to give you diverse citations from the original source books of Ayurveda is to make you realise the various dimensions of a truly holistic system and its benefits in our lives. It is important to know that disintegration of body and mind, as done in modern medicine, is not acceptable to Ayurveda. Psychosomatic ailments and other related disorders are also very recent in the history of modern medicine. But Ayurveda has more profound wisdom than just psychosomatic as here soma affects the psyche and psyche affects the soma. In fact, there is an integral communication in them and only together they make an entire system along with the soul. This latter is the cause of being of the material body made of five elements and provides it the capacity to perform and think. Thinking and performance are not separable. The body or the sharira is inclusive of mind. Mind and body together make that part of a being which disintegrates upon death. Five elements of the body go back to their main pool. Soul, the cause of being, is the continuity. That is why, it is considered as the real self of an individual. When the soul is without body, it is still coded with the karma of that particular individual. It is these codes that are instrumental in deciding about the future of a particular soul.

Karma

Our sages said our ailments are the result of our karma. The karma can be of this life or of previous life or lives. Japa, prayers, meditation and other methods of evoking spiritual energy reduce the bad effects of the past karma. The present karma is in our hands and if we lead a health-oriented life as has been described in this book, we can save ourselves from many health hazards.

Somehow, for the last fifty years, we have been constantly diverting from nature and have created many clashes with it in relation to our body and mind. These clashes have resulted in confusion and chaos in our society and environment.

Human greed has changed our existence considerably. Profit-making organisations and multinationals brainwash people to utilise anti-health products and drugs. Millions of people all over the world have troubles with simple functions of the body like sleep, excretion, and digestion. The modern life-style combined with artificial fertilisers and pesticides, and along with the chemical drugs is resulting in dysfunction of the organisms like kidneys, heart, liver, and pancreas. It is high time that we as individuals learn to save ourselves by awakening our wisdom about our bodies and take our own responsibility.

Pragyaparadha or the Intellectual Error

Unrighteous acts or adharma, whether done by individuals or the community, are due to intellectual error or pragyaparadha. Intellectual error is done due to the lack of sattva. When sattva is diminished and rajas and tamas dominate, the intellect is surrounded by darkness. Sattva by itself is the pure state of intellect and wisdom. In this state of mind, one cannot commit errors. With intellectual errors at administrative and community level, the four common factors to the community are deranged and the whole natural balance is disturbed. The four major factors that affect everybody are air, water, place and time.

Agnivesha asks Lord Atreya in Charaka Samhita (Vimanasthana, III, 20) about the root cause of the derangement of the four factors due to which epidemics arise and destroy the community.

Lord Atreya replied:

The root cause of the derangement of all (air, water, place and time) is unrighteousness or adharma. Adharma also arises due to the misdeeds of the former life or this life but the source of both is intellectual error (pragyaparadha). (This latter is done) when the heads of the country, city, guild and community having transgressed the virtuous path, deal in an unrighteous manner with the people, their officers and subordinates, people of the city and community, and the traders carry this unrighteousness further. Righteousness disappears and the divine powers abandon that place. Seasons get affected and because of this, it does not rain in time or at all or there is abnormal rainfall. Winds do not blow properly, the land is affected, the water reservoirs get dried up and the herbs give up their natural properties and acquire morbidity. The epidemics break out due to polluted contacts and edibles.

From the above citation, we see that the pattern of deterioration in the society has been the same thousands of years. Traders are the multinationals now. They are promoted by various governments for personal gains to sell anti-health products all over the world. We should always awaken our inner wisdom with sattva and should make an effort not to make intellectual errors at any level—family, community or social. If each of us takes the responsibility to fight out adharma and invoke sattva within us, we can avoid intellectual errors. Each one of us is a part of the community and we can stand against adharma of the bigger powers only with knowledge, awakening, unity and strength. Always remember that the products that pollute our environment or ruin our health must be rejected. If all of us do that, there will be an absence of consumers; the big profit making companies will not have any basis to make those products.

Health food stores in Europe used to be separated from the normal food stores. More and more people gradually became aware of the organically grown food and such other things which promote health and energy. Due to that, most normal food stores made a section on health food. With the increasing demand, more and more farmers have started growing food organically. When the demand enhances more, there is depletion in the production of the artificial fertilisers and pesticides. This is a revolution that people can bring. There was something encouraging to that effect I observed in Noida (a satellite town of New Delhi), where I live a part of the year. There are many new restaurants from multinationals selling Americanised junk food. They are struggling to exist and always giving a lot of concessions and special offers. On the contrary, there is a good vegetarian, southern Indian restaurant that has queues of people in front of it during meal times.

As always is the case, some people learn about health awareness on their own whereas there are others who learn the hard way—like getting sick with a serious or chronic ailment. Finally, each one of us is responsible for ourselves and each one of us has an intellect to decide and choose for ourselves. Human freedom lies in the fact that we can decide for our own karma. There is no destiny as such; we are the makers of our own destiny.

Pragyaparadha is in fact the cause of disorders at diverse levels. It is the performance of an unwholesome action that is called pragyaparadha. Unwholesome action is performed due to lack of knowledge and restraint and derangement of memory. These three happen due to rajas and tamas and lack of sattva. Due to lack of sattva, one is not able to distinguish between the soul (eternal) and non-soul (all that is sensuous and non-eternal). Sattva is pure intellect or buddhi and by nature, intellect sees right. It guides us to perform right actions.

In conclusion, to keep good health and to attain longevity, it is absolutely essential to imbibe sattva. It is sattva that guides us to perform wholesome actions and saves us from pragyaparadha.

Importance of Yoga and Sattva in Ayurveda

As is evident from the above description, sattva is of prime importance from Ayurvedic point of view. Sattva is one of the three qualities of mind and it creates equilibrium in rajas (the activity and movement) and tamas (the inactivity and all that which hinders motion). For attaining six dimensional equilibrium, it is essential to imbibe sattva and make an effort to have stillness of mind, compassion, friendship, kindness and generosity.

Methods of yoga are instrumental for integrating sattva in life. Yogasanas, pranayama and japa lead us towards sattva and help attain stillness of mind. Asanas are a part of the therapy for several aches and pains. Pranayama is used for mental and spiritual therapy.

The concept of body in both yoga and Ayurveda is the same. Both these disciplines have fundamentals of Samkhya thought. Body is holy and every effort should be made to keep it in good condition. For an adept of yoga, it is fundamental to have a healthy body in order to concentrate on various meditative practices. The aim of yoga is to achieve liberation from the cycle of birth and death. However the purpose of Ayurveda is to work towards human well-being and to achieve health, happiness and longevity. For detailed description of this theme, you may consult my book—*Patanjali and Ayurvedic Yoga.*

Rhythm of Nature

We need to lead a nature-oriented life and breathe with the rhythm of sun, moon, stars, summer, winter, forest, desert, north, south, and so on. Knowing our surroundings and ourselves well and then adjusting ourselves with the ever-changing dynamic cosmos, is a major step to health. You have seen during the course of this book that Ayurvedic wisdom fundamentally teaches us that we are a part of nature and the functions of our body and mind are linked with the functions of the rest of the cosmos. The whole cosmos is a self-organising whole. Sun rises in the morning, sets in the evening. Weather changes, leaves fall and new leaves appear at the right time. Things do not happen in a haphazard manner in nature. The sun rises gradually and sets the same way. I observe that many people, especially in the West, jump out of their beds in the mornings, go under a shower and dress up very quickly to begin their workday. This is going against the rhythm of nature. This is a shock to the body. Like the cycle of day and night, the rhythm of the body is such that during the night, the srotas or the energy channels of the body gradually come to rest. During the night, they are partially closed and gradually reopen in the morning. Therefore, to jump out of bed and take a shower immediately is being nasty to your body. Let yourself be with the rhythm of nature and do not go against its organisation. The simple practices described in this book like getting up and praying to the sun with some special breathing practices and drinking hot water bring your body and mind gradually into the rhythm of a new day and help imbibe sattvic values.

Ailments and Disorders

There are three kinds of ailments according to Ayurveda: innate, exogenous and psychic.

Innate ailments are those that arise due to imbalance in three doshas— vata, pitta and kapha.

Exogenous ailments are those that arise due to external factors like poisons, polluted air, parasites, bacteria, virus, etc.

Psychic ailments are caused by unfulfilled desires or facing the undesired.

These three kinds of ailments are interconnected and interdependent. An imbalance of the three vital energies not only causes innate disorders related to the doshas but also causes general weakness and lowers the immunity, thus making one vulnerable to external attacks. Similarly, certain kinds of innate disorders when not attended to give rise to or promote psychic ailments. For example, kapha imbalance may lead to depression in certain cases. If kapha vitiation symptoms like heaviness in the body, sweet taste in the mouth, over-salivation, sedentary life-style, over-sleep, etc. are not attended to and they are enhanced by other factors like wet and cold weather, one is liable to get some symptoms of depression. Similarly, with vata vitiation one can get sleep disorders, giving rise to ailments like nervousness, hallucinations, loss and confusion of memory. Pitta imbalance may give rise to excessive and uncontrollable anger.

With different psychic ailments, vital energies lose their balance. For example, if someone is suffering from depression, this person may gradually get kapha disorders as well. Someone who worries excessively and to an abnormal level due to unfulfilled desires or facing the situations that are not pleasant or desirable, may also get vata disorders like sleep disturbances, menstrual problems and constipation. Someone who has an uncontrollable and abnormal anger may also get problems related to the digestive fire, liver, pancreas, etc.

Imbalance of vital energies cause weakness and one becomes liable to various external attacks from bacteria, virus or toxins. Thus, various physical and psychic disorders form a network with each other and you should understand that to find out the root cause of your ailments.

Therapy in Ayurveda

Therapy in Ayurveda is also three-dimensional: rational, mental and spiritual and these three should be applied simultaneously.

Rational therapy is related to drug, exercise, yogasanas and other curative measures like warm baths, enemas and so on.

Mental therapy is to provide mental strength and assurance to the patient that he or she will get all right soon. Mental strength enhances the healing process. When we are sick and are also discouraged, the effect of rational therapy is also slow. Mental therapy should be provided by the physician, friends and family. The sick person can use various methods of yoga and pranayama to enhance the mental strength and promote healing.

Spiritual therapy is very prevalent in India. It is done by prayers, japa, tapa (austarity), pilgrimages, blessings from holy persons, stones, ashes, etc. The fundamental basis of this therapy is to invoke the sattvic and spiritual energy present within us and to channel it for healing. People go to great yogis and sadhus to seek their blessings and bring ceremonious ashes from great temples for their ailing friends or family members. Some ailing persons make a wish to undertake great pilgrimage upon recovery and there are others who pledge to give donations. All these fall in the category of spiritual therapy.

Spiritual therapy is still alive in Southern Europe whereas in Western and Northern Europe it has almost disappeared and most people depend almost exclusively on rational therapy from the allopathic medical system. However, several methods of spiritual therapy from the East are being used by some people whereas others with an exclusively rational approach sneer at these. Recently, in modern medicine, psychotherapy is also being used for people suffering from serious and fatal diseases.

Importance of the three dimensional therapy: In Ayurveda, the body is not considered like a machine as in allopathic system of medicine. Thus, the healing process is also not like a mechanical action where a physician is trying to mend the body machine exclusively at rational level. In Ayurvedic therapeutics, the rational aspect with remedies and other methods is extremely important. In fact, the rational therapy in Ayurveda has a very broad approach as besides the drugs, there are other measures like hot and cold treatments, purification practices, massage, yogic exercises, and detailed instructions about nutrition and specific ways of taking various drugs to avoid their side-effects. Nevertheless, it is extremely important that the patient gets appropriate mental therapy so that his/her mental energy is also diverted to promote the healing process. Spiritual therapy through japa and other methods provide the stillness of mind and invoke the energy from the Self or the soul. This energy is very powerful and it enhances the healing process.

There are several new methods of spiritual therapy like pranic healing, spirit healing, and so on, which are in fact derived from the ancient traditional or shamanistic methods. Some people tend to get fascinated with these methods and use them exclusively, ignoring the rational and mental therapies. This is harmful and in some cases, with prolonged time, the disease may enhance and may become incurable. Therefore, rational therapy is the foremost and the mental and spiritual therapies should be applied simultaneously.

Concept of Drug in Ayurveda

Drug in Ayurveda is that substance which heals as well as establishes equilibrium of the three vital energies. All that which creates imbalance of doshas and leads to creating an ailment is poisonous. The same substance can be drug for one person with a particular disorder and poison for the other. For example, if you have been too long in the hot sun and have sweated too much, you may develop pain in your feet and legs. About ¼ teaspoon of rock salt or ordinary salt in water along with lemon juice and some candy sugar will cure this pain. On the other hand, for someone with hypertension or someone who has symptoms of pitta or kapha vitiation, taking this salty drink will be harmful. Remedies can be as simple as cold milk or chewing a few cloves with dried raisins after meals to treat the problem of stomach acidity. If you are frequently thirsty and have a dry throat again and again, you should drink hot water. There are thousands of very simple remedies which can be made from spices and herbs we use in our Indian cuisine every day. A simple thing like hot water can be preventive and curative in many cases. Since I have mentioned that you should take hot water every morning, I will give below a description of its properties.

Importance of Hot Water

Drinking hot water in the morning is of tremendous importance for good health and longevity. It helps open the energy channels gradually and cleans the alimentary canal. However, if we drink hot tea or some-thing else that is hot, it does not have the same function as drinking hot water. The digestive system has to work to digest the other drinks and water just goes through the system and helps open the energy channels or the srotas. That means, before we put our body to perform various functions, we are waking it up with tenderness and preparing it to take its day's functions gradually. Besides, the water taken on empty stom-ach cleans the digestive tract, ensures proper evacuation and cleans the urinary system.

Persons who suffer from constipation or partial evacuation are cured with drinking hot water. Ayurveda lays a great emphasis on regular and proper evacuation because if some mala (dirt or excrements) re-main inside the body, it rots very quickly and spoils the internal envi-ronment of the body. In fact, persons who suffer from regular constipa-tion or partial evacuation tend to get sleep problems, allergies and skin ailments. According to Ayurveda, the body and mind is a single unity and if one part of the body is dirty, it affects all the physical and mental functions. Through this dirty part, the blood also gets dirty, thus giving rise to allergies and skin ailments. Due to spoilt internal environment, the mind grows restless resulting in sleep disturbances or bad dreams. According to Ayurveda, constipation or partial evacuation gives rise to vata vikriti. Sleep is one of the functions of vata and thus it is affected.

I have described in one of my books that our modern times are vata vitiating. The fast and hectic pace of life, preserved foods and competi-tive lifestyle are all the factors that vitiate vata. Drinking hot water is also a remedy for pacifying vata vitiation. Thus, morning hot water helps us to gain mental and physical balance for the day.

Hot water can be used at other times of the day also to pacify vata vi-tiation. Think of drinking a glass of hot water, preferably cardamom water in the following circumstances:

1. Feeling restless and are unable to concentrate.
2. Feeling tired and are yawning.
3. Have stomach-ache or heaviness in the stomach.
4. Wake up in the middle of the night and are unable to go back to sleep.
5. If you tend to get symptoms of vata vitiation often, drink always hot water whenever you are thirsty.

Complicated remedies for rare diseases may include some rare plants from the upper Himalayas or Iran or Italy or any other part of the world. There are also minerals, special bhasmas (ashes) from various metals and stones and there are also rare products from animals. For Ayurvedic remedies, herbs and minerals are imported from all over the world besides our own tremendous wealth.

Ayurvedic pharmacology is based upon the rasa theory mentioned in Chapter 1 and it is taken care that the drugs are in equilibrium. For example if you are preparing a medicine for treating weak liver and it is bitter (which generally is the case), the bitter rasa is balanced with pungent otherwise it will have a side-effect of vata imbalance. The traditional medicine for cough and cold or phlegm, called Sitopaladi has been described in the Chapter 7. Besides other things, this preparation contains long pepper (pippali), which is very hot in its Ayurvedic qualities. We do need something very 'hot' to get rid of the accumulated phlegm which is a kapha ailment. To make it a balanced preparation without side-effects, candy sugar (mishri) and cardamom are added into this preparation.

Thus, we see that Ayurveda is a highly advanced system of health and healing. It is the result of hard work of thousands of years and a tremendous amount of research on nature and its ways of functioning. It is time that we wake up to our priceless heritage and utilise it for the benefit of humanity.

Many people think that all herbal medicines or remedies made from natural substances do not have any side-effects. It is a grossly mistaken notion. There are many highly poisonous plants. Dhatura's flowers are offered to Lord Shiva, but this is highly poisonous. It is used in Ayurvedic medicines but its daily dose should be limited to 50 mg per day. If taken in higher doses, besides the negative effects on your eyes and heart, it results in loss of memory. There are instances when it's frequent and over-use has caused people to forget their own name for a long duration of time. The idea to state all this is to make you realise that Ayurveda is an absolutely scientific system which provides the effect of drugs in totality along with their doses, frequency and other allied prescriptions.

Ayurvedic wisdom about drugs is tremendous and one needs a proper study of this system in its totality to understand and use them in a correct manner. Ayurvedic drugs are not tried on rats or other laboratory animals but human beings have been using them successfully since eternity. We need not waste money on doing experiments on animals with Ayurvedic remedies. This is ridiculous that the remedies which we have been using for many generations and we grew up seeing their healing results should be subjected to scrutiny. This shows a lack of confidence in our indigenous methods of health and healing. There are no reasons to believe that the western norms for science and medicine are absolute.

It is observed that some scientists and doctors trained in modern science and medicine get interested in Ayurveda but do not understand it properly as they do not devote enough time to study the extensive wisdom of Ayurveda. Some of them condemn it as being too complicated and unscientific to cover up their ignorance. There are others who get so fascinated with this limitless wisdom that leave behind all to devote their lives for the research and development of Ayurveda. Giving an example of the former category, once I attended a lecture by a professor in Delhi on herbal medicine. This person was doing clinical trials with some Ayurvedic plant products. He started his lecture by showing a slide of Lord Hanuman carrying a little hillock and said that when Hanuman, being a god could not recognise the Sanjivani plant and had to carry the whole hillock, how can we human beings do that. The conclusion of this elderly professor with many foreign degrees was that Ayurveda is too complicated. Many of you know the epic of Ramayana. Hanuman was known for his supernatural powers and his extraordinary physical strength. But he was not an Ayurvedic physician. When Lakshaman fainted during the war between Rama and Ravana, Vaidya Sushen was called. Sushen knew exactly what plant was required to revive Lakshaman, where it is found, how the medicine was prepared from this plant and what were the doses to be given. And all of us know that Sushen did succeed in reviving Lakshaman with his wisdom of Ayurveda. Hanuman as god helped him to make the herb available with supernatural strength but the knowledge of Ayurveda was not his domain.

There are thousands of Ayurvedic remedies which have been used in Indian homes since eternity. I call it 'grandmother's tradition'. It was either an elderly person in the family or in the village who passed on the secrets of remedies to cure common ailments. Besides the remedies, there was also the wisdom about other aspects of treatment such as nutrition, exercise, mental state, massage, oil treatment, thermal therapy, etc. Ayurvedic physicians took care of more serious ailments which ordinary human beings could not handle. A traditional vaidya collects the herbs herself/himself, makes powders, extracts, remedies and other allied things. He/she is capable of identifying plants and in certain cases when herbs are bought, they are recognised with various characteristics including their smell and taste.

The old and traditional methods are getting lost with the rapid modernisation and what we need to do is to reorganise our ancient wisdom and spread it through modern techniques. We have to take care that there is some standardisation by the experts and with simplicity and precision we should bring the knowledge of remedies to people. As you know, there are so many aspects of Ayurveda than just the remedies, and other instructions like nutrition and lifestyle should also be given. To revive all this, there is a great need to bring Ayurvedic education to our schools as well as in medical colleges.

Vitamins and Minerals

Many times I have been asked about the importance of minerals and vitamins in Ayurveda. The answer is simple. With a large variety of substances we consume in Ayurveda and the importance of rasayanas, there is no chance that we can have a dearth of vitamins and minerals. Besides, in Ayurveda, in case of deficiency, specific diets and drugs are prescribed. According to Ayurvedic wisdom, the extraction of individual chemicals and their intake is not recommended. For example, in case of deficiency of iron and vitamin C, amala is recommended. For calcium deficiency, sesames seeds and oil are recommended besides cheese and other milk products. Intake of vitamins in pure form as prescribed in allopathy enhances the metabolism in the body and from Ayurvedic point of view, it will vitiate pitta and vata.

Is Ayurveda Expensive?

Ayurveda has become very popular in the West during the last few years. There are several kinds of offers—massage being the most popular. Many take a very limited meaning of Ayurveda as it was revealed in one of the advertisements I saw in Germany. It said something like this:

AYURVEDA: Enjoy the treatment of Maharajas for looking young and beautiful. Now you can enjoy the treatments that only Maharajas could afford in the former times.

This indeed shows a very wrong notion of Ayurveda. Ayurveda is science of life as the name also indicates. It is an integral part of Indian life and culture. When a housewife adds roasted cumin in yoghurt or adds garlic in the dals (lentils), it is Ayurveda. The other day I asked for peanuts at my grocer's shop. His little son was helping his father at the shop. He said to me, "You want to eat peanuts in this heat?" This is also Ayurvedic wisdom. You get a pimple on your face and your mother or an aunt tells you to eat some neem leaves or karelas (bitter gourd); that is also the basic wisdom of Ayurveda. Ayurveda is how to preserve life in its optimum conditions, how to enhance lifespan and how to rejuvenate oneself, how to prevent ailments and when they are there, how to treat them. There are hundreds of things around us that are low cost and can help us tremendously to regain our strength and enhance our energy. Feeling tired? Go to your kitchen and take half a teaspoon of powdered cumin everyday for a few days or make a tea with big cardamom, cinnamon and clove. Or else make tea with basil (tulsi), ginger, pepper and cardamom (small).

The other aspect of Ayurveda is that to treat a disease you may need a very specific medicine and plants for that medicine may come from the high Himalayas or Italy, Greece or Turkey and your medicine is made of numerous exclusive plants; in that case it will be expensive.

Coming back to massage and 'Maharaja treatment', the important part is the application of oil that provides strength to the body and makes it shock resistant. I have given you the ways and methods of doing it yourself. That is absolutely false that only Maharajas could afford this treatment in olden times. When I was a child, every morning, a masseur couple came to our house. That was an extended family. The masseuse massaged the women of the family and the masseur massaged the men. Every third or fourth day, each person had his or her turn. Besides that, the massage is also family culture. I have described this kind of familial massage in my book—*Ayurveda, A Way of Life*.

Health and Joie de Vivre in Ayurveda

Since body is not considered like a mechanical system in Ayurveda, the concept of health is not merely the correct functioning of the body machine. Health is considered as the optimum state of being with high level of mental and physical energy. It is also meant to have tough body resistance and to have the ability to fight back negative forces like infections, fatigue, effect of aging, accidents etc. Geriatrics is an important part of Ayurveda and so is rejuvenation in the sense of enhancing energy levels and strengthening the immune system. Human beings are supposed to take care of themselves intensively (as you must have realised from this whole book) even without being sick. Thus, prevention of all kinds of ailments and disorders are of high priority in Ayurveda.

There is a great emphasis on human happiness in Ayurveda. The technical term used for this is 'prasannachitta' (a happy state of mind). Sushruta has used this term and it is said that for keeping good health and for healing in case of ailments, a mental state of inner joy and happiness plays a great role. It enhances the process of healing. In fact, this concept for health and healing was widely used also by the ancient Greeks. The Greeks made great health resorts that included many art forms including big theatres and with many diverse modes of entertainment. Music and theatre were particularly used for healing.

According to Ayurveda, dissatisfaction (asantosha) is the root cause of many ailments. A mental state of dissatisfaction is the tamasic state of mind. It brings the ojas down and gives rise to fatigue. Individuals who usually have a disposition to be dissatisfied look fatigued and unhealthy. They grow old fast and when they get sick, the recovery time is long. Therefore, make effort to keep yourself happy and satisfied in pursuit of good health. Keep contented and in troubled times, always console yourself by saying that things could have been even worse.

Health care in Ayurveda is not at all through tears as this ancient wisdom has many secrets of enhancing sexual pleasure and joys of the pallet. In ancient texts there is a description of different kinds of wines, beers and alcohols. Unfortunately, these are not made any more and it seems that this wisdom is lost forever. It is said in Ayurveda that one should take a moderate quantity of good quality wine or beer with food. One should not drink on an empty stomach and neither excessively. Tobacco did not exist in India at the time of Charaka but there were many other plants which were used for smoking. Moderate and ceremonious smoking is recommended for the sake of relaxation.

As I have mentioned in the first Chapter of the book, 'Virility, Sexuality and Fertility' are one of the eight parts of Ayurveda. There are many methods to enhance sexual energy. Different aphrodisiacs are used in specific cases. For example, there are some to enhance the quality and quantity of sexual secretions. There are others that are used to enhance the sexual urge and vigour. There are yet another category of aphrodisiacs to enhance potency. There are methods for prolonging the sexual duration for men and shortening the sexual duration for women to bring coordination in the sexual act for two partners. There are methods to treat impotency and other sexual problems. I have given some of these methods in my three books: *Ayurveda for life— Nutrition, Sexual Energy and Healing, The Kamasutra for Women* and *Companionship and Sexuality.*

Some Experiences with Ayurveda

Vyadhi or the ailments are a part of our existence. From time to time, all of us need medical help. According to Ayurveda, body heals itself if we have an ailment that is not too serious and is curable. The role of the physician and the medication is to enhance the process of healing and lessen the suffering of the patient. Thus, the process of healing is normally gradual and the aim is to get rid of infection if any and bring the body back to equilibrium (state of prakriti). One should not suppress the symptoms of the ailment as is done with alchemy and allopathic drugs. Take the example of a simple ailment like common cold. There are allopathic drugs that claim quick relief from the cold. The

186

danger is that after a quick relief from the cold, the phlegm may get accumulated in the sinuses or the remains of the infection may get accumulated there and you may get frequent attacks of the cold thereafter. From Ayurvedic point of view, all those methods should be used that can throw out the phlegm one way or another. Therefore, warm measures are taken, inhalation is done, teas hot in their Ayurvedic nature are taken and preparation like chickpea flour is taken to reduce the formation of the phlegm (see the details of curing common cold in the last chapter). Thus, every effort is made to throw out the accumulated phlegm and to stop the formation of new phlegm. With this therapy, after you are cured, you feel healthy and not weak.

Experience with Ayurvedic treatment is different than with allopathic treatment. Most allopathic treatments leave you with the imbalance of the three vital energies and you feel tired after the therapy. Many traditional persons in India who take allopathic treatment often complain that the medications give rise to vata and pitta imbalance. Then there are series of allopathic drugs used for hypertension, sleep disorders and other neurological disorders that also give rise to kapha imbalance. This is the reason that many people who take allopathic treatment for a long time, get other disorders gradually and can never get back to normal again. This is an extremely valuable contribution of Ayurveda, that it aims at purifying and balancing the system along with curing the disorder. The Ayurvedic treatment does not leave behind complications and new ailments to deal with. In fact, in Ayurveda, the aim is to treat the person and not exclusively the ailment.

I have personal experiences and exceptional cases of treatment done by other Ayurvedic physicians and it may be interesting for you to obtain this first hand information. It is important to know that there are many disorders that modern medicine cannot treat whereas Ayurveda has a wealth of wisdom for them. I do not mean to condemn the system of modern medicine. We have excellent diagnostic equipments and wonderful methods to deal with emergencies. The ancient methods of Ayurvedic surgery are now lost and the methods of surgery in modern medical systems are unparalleled. What is not right in the modern medical system is overuse and indiscriminate use of drugs. We do not need all those drugs to cure our minor problems and to pollute our systems with them.

The fevers in Delhi: For part of the year I live in the Delhi area and fever is a speciality of this highly polluted part of the country. During the change of weather and around the time of monsoons, every third person is suffering from what they call viral fever. Most people go to doctors and get antibiotics and analgesics. There are new and more resistant viruses every year and each time they have their peculiar symptoms. Once I got an attack of one of the nasty viruses in the beginning of winter. The fever was very high and very persistent and it did not reduce with my bitter mixtures and diverse teas. My housekeeper panicked and brought some analgesics that I refused to take. With the third day of high fever, I had lost my capacity to treat myself and was confused. The fever did not come down below 40^0 C (104^0 F). I did not have a special Ayurvedic medicine for fever, which of course I made after this incident (see Chapter 7 for this remedy). I was doing spiritual therapy and the effect of the mantras and the fever together, I got the revelation of the medicine I needed. That was Giloye (Guduchi in Sanskrit and *Tinospora cordifolia* in Latin). My housekeeper Govind, who is from a village in Bihar knew how to make a preparation from Giloye. He cooked the stem in water and took out the extract from it, mixed sugar with this extract to mask the bitter taste. He gave me a glass full of it and I drank. In three–four hours, the fever came down to little more than normal. I felt good and well. The next day the second dose brought the fever to normal and I was absolutely fine.

I asked the young man how did he know about making this medicine. He explained to me that in his village, people take it as a rasayana.

The interesting part of the story is that during the following month after this incident, I heard many people talk about this awful virus that gave high fever, which could not be cured with any of the prevalent allopathic drugs.

Giloye is a climber and its leaves resemble that of beetle. It is a very fast growing plant and it takes its nourishment in such an aggressive way that the plants growing around it in a garden either die or fair badly. For that reason, I had this plant removed from my garden but had not de-rooted it. The plant was cut from the ground and up to the two storeys of the house. Some parts of it remained hung from the top floor. It did dry up but apparently it was still alive as during the monsoons, it started sending fine roots like silk threads towards the ground in search of food. Leaves were coming out from the stem which was hanging in the air. Apparently, it got enough nourishment from the humid air of that season. I felt that with the same aggressively, this plant did wonders to treat fever.

My idea to tell you this story is to show you how powerful nature is and how wise our ancestors were to study the diversity of this universe and find oneness in all phenomena. There are thousands of plants like that in nature that can help us in various ways and bless us with health and happiness.

Memory and creativity: During recent years, there has been much talk in Indian media that scientists have made a tablet from Brahmi plant that promotes memory. Brahmi (*Cintella asiatica*) is classified as **an intellect promoting** plant since eternity in Ayurveda. This is a paradox in India that this ancient Indian wisdom is now advertised as something newly found in the medical sciences. The wisdom of those sages, who told us about the wonderful qualities of Brahmi thousands of years ago, does not need validation from modern scientists with modern equipment and after torturing the laboratory animals.

In Ayurveda, there are several plants which are used together to enhance the brain functions and to rejuvenate the brain. They not only promote memory but also enhance concentration and creativity. With many years of research, I have made several combinations of brain rejuvenating products to enhance diverse functions. One of the very amazing plants belongs to the lavender family and is imported from Persia (Iran). This plant is called 'Broom of the brain'. This name is indeed very amusing but has a great pharmacological significance. It is specially given to people who feel heaviness in head and according to Ayurveda, have kapha imbalance and blockades in the head region. When given to such patients, they actually hear 'strange sounds and some movements' in their heads; hence the name of the plant. The effect of this plant is that it gives relief through purification. It frees the head region from excessive kapha that apparently blocks the brain functions.

According to my experience, brain-rejuvenating products can also be used for some mental disorders as well as some neurological disorders. By strengthening and promoting brain functions, we can alleviate the fundamental weakness of this organism that initially becomes the cause of these disorders in many cases. The brain rejuvenating products can be successfully used to promote learning and to enhance work-efficiency for students and other people who have to work a lot with their brains

Remedies for arthritis: Arthritis is a vata ailment. Rheumatoid arthritis is a vata-kapha ailment. These two can be treated successfully with Ayurvedic methods. The treatment is also cost effective. But as has been evident from this book, Ayurvedic treatment is holistic and it also demands a change in your life-style as well as your thinking process. These two are very powerful; they can become the cause of ailments and can also heal them. I have seen some exceptional and very advanced cases of arthritis being cured by Arya Vaidya Sala from Kottakkal, Kerala. These people have also opened a centre in Delhi now.

Treatment of infertility: Infertility can be due to many diverse reasons and all cases are not curable. But in many cases, the Ayurvedic purification practices, intake of rasayanas and some specific aphrodisiacs can treat it. There are aphrodisiacs that promote the sperm count and enhance the quality of the sperms. Vitiation of vata can cause infertility in both the sexes. Massage, warm treatments like vapour baths and fomentations and enemas are essential to treat vata imbalance. Vata hinders the implantation of the foetus in case of women. Thus, despite fertilisation, they are unable to conceive.

I have seen many successful cases of the treatment of infertility by able vaidyas and have also myself treated some cases with very simple methods. Remember that most people turn to Ayurvedic or other alternative methods after they have tried their best with the allopathic treatment and they have been declared incapacitated to have children.

Treatment of mountain sickness: I was travelling in Laddhak and we were going in a bus to the highest mountain pass in the world—the Khardungla pass (5385 meter/17770 feet). We were very close to the pass when we all had to get down from the bus, as a part of the road was broken. We walked about 100 meters and an elderly man got sick

190

due to the height and the effort he had to make to walk. I gave him a preparation made of lemons and some spices. He felt a relief immediately and the curious fellow passengers asked me about the magical stuff I gave him. It was nothing but a lemon pickle which was made in Indian homes in the former times. This preparation is made with lot of spices, particularly with ajwain. I researched and added a few more things in this age-old recipe to treat the stomach problems, indigestion, dry throat due to vata and the mountain sickness. I have given this recipe in my book on *Ayurvedic Food Culture and Recipes*.

There are hundreds of things like that which are simple and easy to prepare and all the products are available around us. We can treat ourselves in a very simple and easy manner which is also economical and save ourselves from the ill effects of the treatment with chemicals.

Vaidyas in Modern India

Vaidya Brihaspati Dev Triguna in New Delhi near Nizamudin railway station sees 200 patients a day. He sees your pulse and tells you in a dramatic manner what your problems are. Whenever I need help, I go to him. From time to time, I met patients there who told me the tales of their deadly disease and how Triguna ji's treatment made them live once again more or less a normal life. Triguna ji and his family work in the traditional style and that means that the vaidyas are also pharmacologists and pharmacists and they provide patients with medicines made by them. Besides, the combinations and proportions of drugs differ for each patient.

We have many sincere and able vaidyas throughout the country but there is no dearth of quacks as well. Thus, we should be very careful while choosing our physician. Charaka expresses in Sutrasthana his strong opinion about the quacks and says:

It is better to self-immolate than to be treated by an ignorant physician. A physician should possess the following qualities— excellence in theoretical knowledge, extensive practical experience, dexterity and cleanliness. The physician who possesses the knowledge of the four aspects—cause, symptom, cure and prevention of the disease—is the best.

A physician should be friendly and compassionate towards the sick and should not be greedy.

Thus, we should be very careful in our choice of the physician. On the part of the patient, he or she should be obedient and follow the prescriptions about diet, medication and allied things for treatment.

Various Steps of Treatment

With Ayurvedic wisdom, we can treat many of our minor disorders on our own. As you have learnt, many small but nagging ailments are due to an imbalance of the three principal energies of the body. An imbalance can give rise to a series of troubles and by treating the imbalance, we can also cure a number of troubles. Constipation, dry throat, disturbed sleep and nervousness are vata related disorders. When we become aware of that and take measures to bring vata to equilibrium, we are also able to heal several of these disorders simultaneously. Thus, the emphasis should be on maintaining the equilibrium of the doshas.

If you are unable to cure yourself despite doing all to gain the equilibrium of doshas, it could mean that you have an external attack or something else that is pathological in your body. In that state, you need the help of an able physician who treats you with holistic methods. Along with the treatment, you need to take care of your diet and way of life. During the time of healing, you need a diet that can be easily digested and is nourishing. You need more rest to enable your body to heal rapidly. Besides, you need to use your mental and spiritual power for healing yourself. What is extremely important is that you keep courage and have confidence in your healing power. Fear is tamas and it is an enemy of the process of healing. The sattva state of mind enhances the process of healing. Forget about all your problems and concentrate your mental and spiritual energy to bring back your body to its natural state of health—prakriti.

The third state of being unhealthy is with a serious sickness or an accident or the effect of a poison. This category of ailment requires a long-term treatment and you need to have both courage and patience. Like in the above case, you need to focus your mental and physical energies on the process of healing. To treat a long-term sickness, perhaps you will have to take some strong medicines which may also have side-effects. If you are being treated in a hospital with allopathic methods, request your physician to put you on some mild kind of medication and on a low dose. Use your wisdom of Ayurveda and take appropriate healing herbs and rasayanas to enhance the process of recovery.

Unfortunately, there are diseases which are totally or almost incurable. In such cases, try not to put yourself or your loved ones in a situation where one has to hang between life and death. From Ayurvedic point of view, such patients should be kept happy and should be given whatever they desire. They should be kept in a pleasant environment so that they are able to attain a 'good death'.

A Timely and Good Death

There is no concept of a 'good death' in allopathic medicine. Death is considered as a failure of the medical profession. But in Charaka Samhita, there is an extensive description of death. In fact, in our traditional homes, it is considered very important to feel good and peaceful at the last moments of one's life. It reminds me of an incident of several years ago. One morning my milkman came to me with some medical reports and a question related to the ailment of his father. He told me that his father was very sick, was in a hospital where treatment was awfully expensive and despite all this, his father wanted to get out of there. He wanted me to advise him on what to do. I looked at the reports and his father was suffering from throat cancer. I suggested to the milkman to have his father out of the hospital and keep him at home and to give him whatever he feels like eating. Basically, the family should make every effort to keep him happy and to help him attain a pleasant death. The milkman and his family brought their father home and tried to keep him happy as much as they could. The father was also smoking his usual beedies (Indian cigarettes rapped in a special leaf) and demanded his favourite dishes. The milkman told me that his father felt much better than when he was in the hospital and showed an improvement in his condition. He lived several months longer than the doctors had estimated.

Agnivesha asked Lord Atreya in Charaka Samhita (Vimanasthanam, III, 37-38) the following question:

O Lord, when people have undetermined lifespan, how there is timely or untimely death?

Lord Atreya replied—O Agnivesha, listen. An axle fitted in a vehicle that is endowed with all the qualities continue to function and perishes in time by depreciation of its normal limit; similarly, the lifespan in a body of a person having strong

193

constitution and managed properly gets its end and loss of its normal limit. Such death is known as timely.

The same axel gets destroyed on the way due to over-load, uneven road, want of road, breaking of wheels, defects in vehicle or driver, separation of the bolt, non-lubrication and throwing about. Similarly, the lifespan comes to an end in the middle due to over-exertion, diet not in accordance with agni, irregular meals, complicated body postures, over-indulgence in sexuality, company of ignoble persons, suppression of impelled urges, non-suppression of suppressible urges, infliction with organism, poisonous winds and fire, injury and avoidance of food and medicaments. Such death is termed as untimely. Similarly, death occurred due to faulty management in cases of fever etc., is also untimely.

The essence of this book is that we should make every effort to keep ourselves healthy, peaceful and satisfied. The aim of life should also be to achieve a good and peaceful end to it. We should do many things for that along with bringing sattvic thoughts in our daily life. We should invest generously in terms of effort, time and money to promote our health and to preserve it well as long as possible. We should not forget that the first priority of life is life itself and when that is gone, everything else is meaningless. It is the first duty or dharma (svadharma) to take care of ourselves and to work towards the well being of our body and mind. Body is the temple of soul; it should be kept clean and healthy.

Rejuvenation of Ayurveda

It is a pity that our ancient wisdom is not put to practice, as it should be. The British rulers did not believe in our indigenous system and our government who has inherited the legacy has still not attained freedom from the British in policy making. Government policies after independence have harmed the traditional medicine tremendously as under the garb of modernisation, the indigenous systems were made to appear primitive and non-scientific. Folks developed complexes about their traditional values being inferior to the modern methods of curing ailments. Gradually, with the revival of the alternative methods of healing the world over, Ayurveda is not only resurrect and rejuvenated in India, also its wisdom is spreading everywhere in the world. I will not use the expression—*revival of Ayurveda* in Indian context, as this rich tradition was never dead. It was and still is thriving in Indian homes. Only it was ignored and put aside by a small section of the society in urban India.

Om Shanti

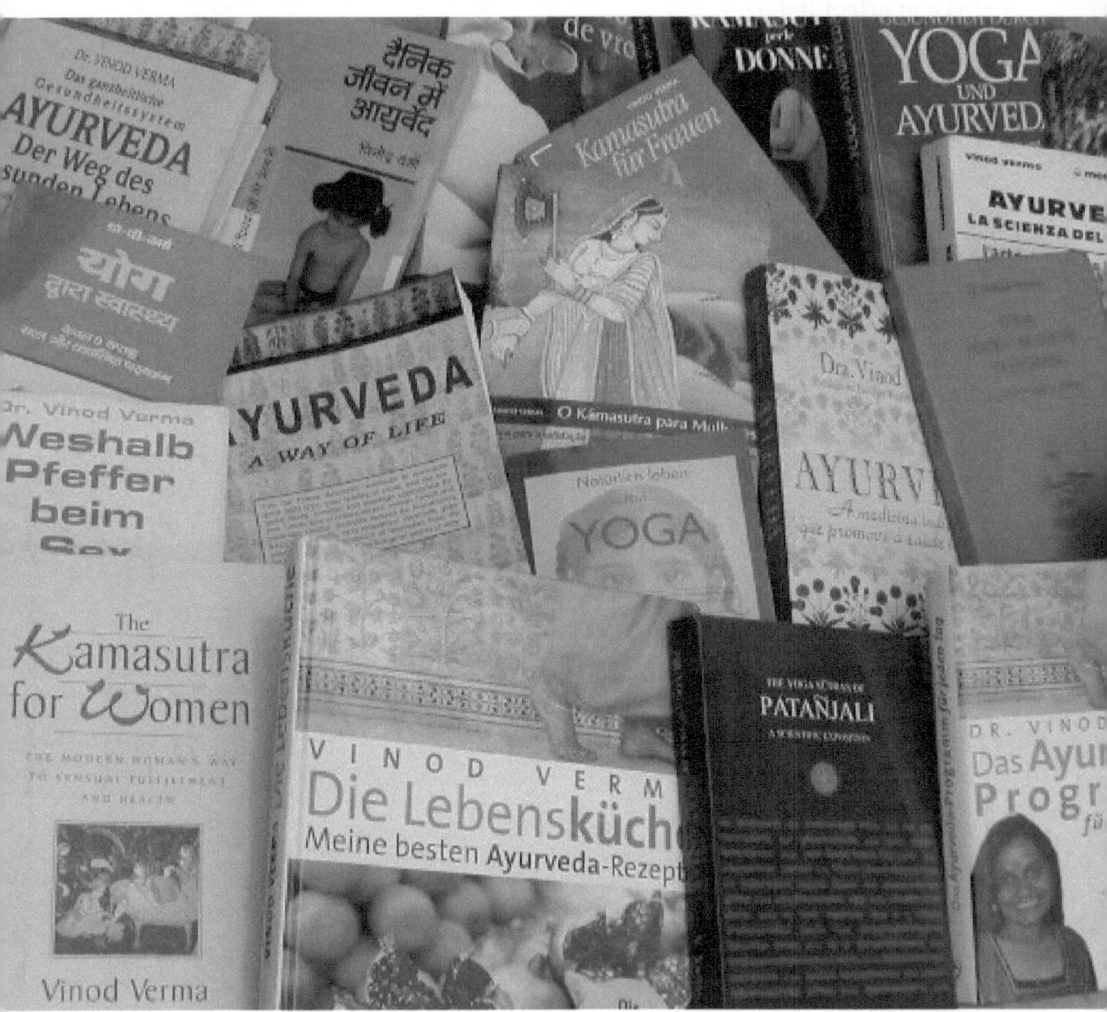

About the Author

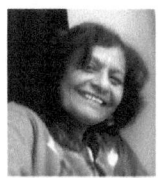 Along with a doctorate degree in reproduction biology in India, Dr. Verma studied Neurobiology in Paris University and obtained a second doctorate. She pursued advanced research at the National Institutes of Health, Bethesda (USA) and the Max-Planck Institute in Freiburg, Germany. At the peak of her career in medical research in a pharmaceutical company in Germany, she realised that the modern approach to health care is basically fragmented and non-holistic. Besides, we are directing all our efforts and resources to cure disease rather than maintaining health. In response, Dr. Verma founded The New Way Health Organisation (NOW) in 1986 to spread the message of holistic living, preventive methods for health care and to promote the use of mild medicine and various self-help therapeutic measures.

Dr. Verma grew up with a strong familial tradition of Ayurveda with a grandmother who had enormous Ayurvedic wisdom and was a gifted healer. She has studied Ayurveda in the traditional Guru-shishya style with Acharya Priya Vrat Sharma of the Benares Hindu University for 23 years.

Dr. Verma is an ardent researcher and is working hard to compile the living tradition of Ayurveda and spread it in the world through her books and other activities. She has published twenty three books on yoga, Ayurveda, Women and Companionship. The books are published in various languages of the world. Besides, she has published numerous scientific articles. Several other books are in preparation. She lectures extensively, teaches in Europe for several months a year, trains students at her two centres in India and gives radio and television programmes. A film on Ayurveda with her was made by German television in 1995 and was shown in 100 countries, in 130 languages. It was the first film on Ayurveda.

Dr. Verma has founded Charaka School of Ayurveda to train interested people with genuine Ayurvedic education so that they can further impart the knowledge of Ayurvedic way of life and save people from becoming a victim of charlatanry in Ayurveda. She is doing several research projects on medicinal plants and their combination in the form of remedies. She is the founder and chairperson of *The Ayurveda Health Organisation*, which is a charitable trust for distributing and promoting Ayurvedic remedies and yoga therapy in rural areas of India. She does regular lectures and workshops for school children in the rural and remote areas of Himalayas to promote wisdom of traditional science and medicine. Dr. Verma gives seminars, lectures and teaches in the *Charaka School of Ayurveda* with guru-shishya tradition.

Dr. Vinod Verma's Publications

1. *Patanjali's Yoga Sutra: A Scientific Exposition* (Published in English, Hindi and German).
2. *Ayurveda for Inner Harmony: Nutrition, Sexual Energy and Healing* (Published in English, German, Italian, French, Romanian and Hindi).
3. *Ayurveda a Way of Life* (Published in English, German, Italian, French, Spanish, Czech, Greek, Portuguese, Slovenian and Hindi).
4. *The Kamasutra for Women* (Published in English [America and India], German, French, Dutch, Romanian, Italian, Portuguese, Slovenian Hindi and Malayalam).
5. *Stress-free Work with Yoga and Ayurveda* (Published in German, English [America and India] and Hindi).
6. *Patanjali and Ayurvedic Yoga* (Published in English, German and Hindi).
7. *Programming Your Life with Ayurveda* (Published in German, French, English, Slovenian and Czech).
8. *Ayurvedic Food Culture and Recipes* (Published in English, German, Czech and Hindi).
9. *Yoga: A Natural Way of Being* (Published in English, German, French, Italian and Hindi).
10. *Companionship and Sexuality: Based on Ayurveda and the Hindu tradition* (Published in English and German).
11. *Natural Glamour: The Ayurveda Beauty Book* (Published in German, Spanish and English)
12. *Losing and Maintaining Weight with Ayurveda and Yoga* (Published in English, Slovenian and German).
13. *The Timeless Wisdom of Ayurveda: A Scientific Exposition* (Published in English and German)
14. *Prakriti and Pulse: The Two Mysteries of Ayurveda* (Published in German)
15. *Good Food for Dogs: Vegetarian nourishment based on Ayurvedic wisdom* (Published in German and English)
16. *Diet for Losing Weight* (published in German and English)
17. *Aum: The Eternal Energy* (Published in German and English)
18. *Pulse Diagnose in Chinese and Ayurvedic Medicine* (co-author for TCM Dr. Florian Ploberger) (published in German)
19. *Shiva's Secrets for Health and Longevity* (published in German and English)
20. *Healing Hands: The Ayurvedic Massage workbook* (published in English)
21. *Prevention of Dementia* (published in German and English)

22. *Ayurveda for Dogs* (published in German and English)
23. Numerology: Based on the Vedic Tradition (published in English and Slovenian)

The Charaka School of Ayurveda and Patanjali Yogadarshana Society (Himalayan Centre)

The Charka School of Ayurveda (CSA) has been founded by Dr. Vinod Verma to spread the genuine classical tradition as well as the living tradition of Ayurveda in the world for promoting healthy living and preventing ailments. Its aim is to teach people a healthy lifestyle which enhances immunity and vitality and enables them to live a life with an optimum level of energy. For minor ailments, people should be capable of using home remedies, appropriate physical and mental exercises and nutrition.

CSA aims to bring genuine and practical aspects of Ayurveda to people and save them from Americanised and Europeanised distorted versions of Ayurveda and other forms of charlatanry that do more harm than good.

To achieve this purpose, CSA trains students from all over the world who can further spread the message of Ayurvedic lifestyle and help people with genuine massages, purification practices, nutrition and other practical aspects of Ayurveda. The school is in association with the most learned persons of Ayurveda in India and several exclusive persons involved in health education in Europe.

The object of Patanjali Yogadarshana Society is to spread the message of Patanjali in the world. The wisdom of the Yoga Sutras is not only beneficial for the yogis but also for our day-to-day normal life. Its aim is to enhance *sattva* or the inner stillness and peace in the world as well as in the individual minds. With years of research on Yoga and Ayurveda, Dr. Verma has founded the Ayurvedic Yoga and has written a book on the subject.

Lectures, Seminars and Training Programmes

To get detailed information on the Charaka School of Ayurveda as well as our other programmes in India and Europe, visit our website or contact us by email.

The New Way Health Organisation .NOW.

A-130, Sector 26, Noida 201301, U.P., India

Tel. 0091 (0)120 2527820 or (0) 9873704205 or (0)9412224820

www.ayurvedavv.com and www.drvinodverma.com
Contact at: ayurvedavv@yahoo.com

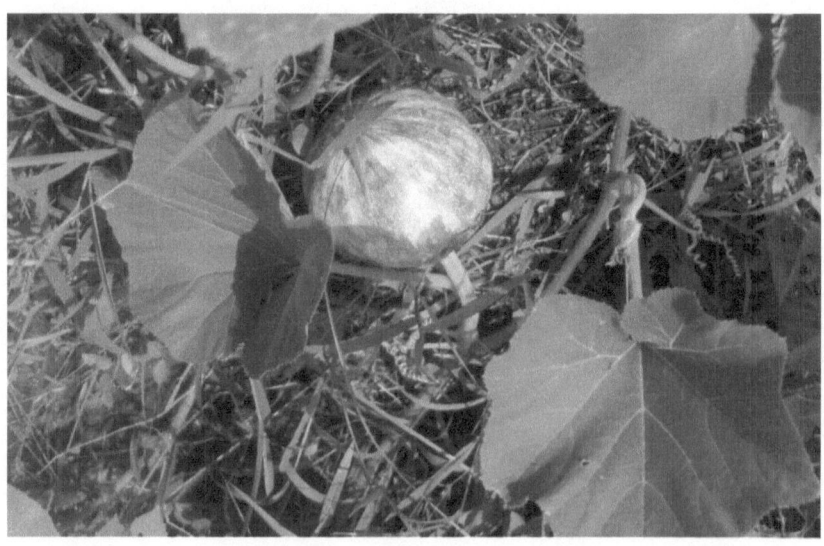

Himalayan Centre

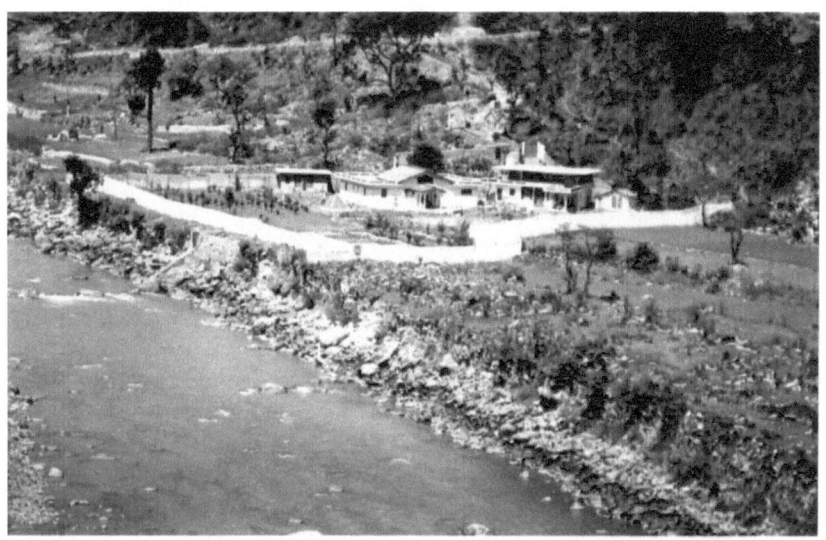

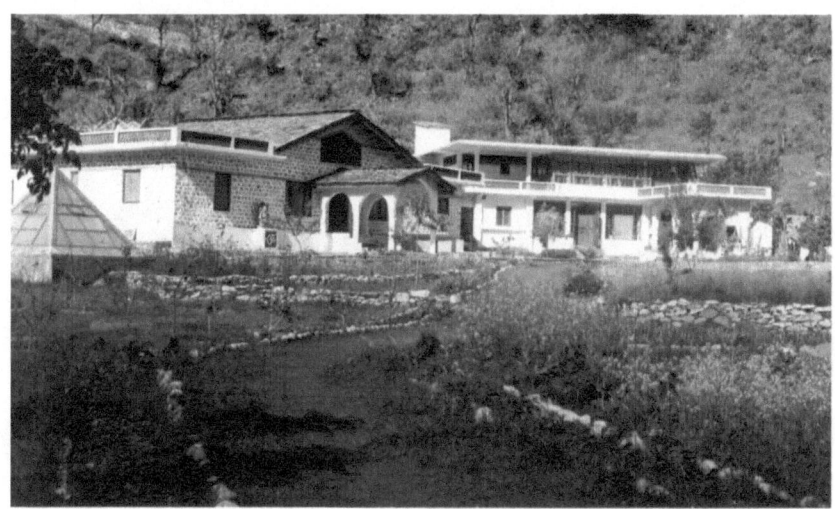

www.ingramcontent.com/pod-product-compliance
Lightning Source LLC
Chambersburg PA
CBHW050443290526
45786CB00006B/2147